T0203387

Clinics in Developmental Medicine

THE PLACENTA AND NEURODISABILITY
2ND EDITION

Clinics in Developmental Medicine

The Placenta and Neurodisability

2nd edition

Edited by

IAN CROCKER
Maternal and Fetal Health Research Centre,
Institute of Human Development
University of Manchester, UK

MARTIN BAX
Emeritus Reader in Child Health, Imperial College
London, UK

2015
Mac Keith Press

Managing Director: Ann-Marie Halligan
Production Manager and Commissioning Editor: Udoka Ohuonu
Project Management: Lumina Datamatics

First published in this edition in 2015

British Library Cataloguing-in-Publication data
A catalogue record for this book is available from the British Library

Cover design: Karl Hunt

ISBN: 978-1-909962-53-8

Typeset by Lumina Datamatics, Chennai, India

Printed by Imprint Digital Limited, Rickmansworth, UK

Mac Keith Press is supported by Scope

CONTENTS

AUTHORS' APPOINTMENTS

Kathryn Abel Professor of Psychological Medicine, University of Manchester; Honorary Consultant Psychiatrist, Manchester Mental Health & Social Care Trust, Manchester, UK

Matthew Allin Honorary Senior Lecturer, Institute of Psychiatry, King's College London, UK

Martin Bax Emeritus Reader in Child Health, Imperial College London, UK

Valentina Brusati Specialist Surgeon in Obstetrics and Gynaecology, Department of Women, Mothers and Neonates, Buzzi Children's Hospital; Institute of Clinical Specialisation, Milan, Italy

Irene Cetin Head of Department of Mother and Child, Hospital Luigi Sacco; Director Giorgio Pardi Centre for Fetal Research Department of Biomedical and Clinical Sciences, University of Milan, Italy

Jayne Charnock Post-Doctoral Research Associate, Maternal and Fetal Health Research Centre, Institute of Human Development, University of Manchester, UK

Ian Crocker Senior Scientist/Lecturer, Maternal and Fetal Health Research Centre, Institute of Human Development, University of Manchester, UK

Michelle Desforges Post-Doctoral Research Associate, Maternal and Fetal Health Research Centre, Institute of Human Development, University of Manchester; Manchester Academic Health Sciences Centre, UK

Emma Ingram Clinical Research Fellow, Maternal and Fetal Health Research Centre, Institute of Human Development, University of Manchester, UK

Catherine James   Clinical Research Fellow, Maternal and Fetal
                         Medicine, Institute for Women's Health,
                         University College London, UK

Ed Johnstone   Clinical Senior Lecturer, Institute of Human
                         Development, University of Manchester, UK

Gil Mor   Professor of Obstetrics, Gynaecology and
                         Reproductive Sciences, School of Medicine,
                         Yale University, Connecticut, USA

Karin Nelson   Scientist Emeritus, National Institute of
                         Neurological Disorders and Stroke, National
                         Institutes of Health, Maryland, USA

Donald Peebles   Chair and Head of the Research Department
                         of Maternal Fetal Medicine, University College
                         London; Honorary Consultant in Maternal Fetal
                         Medicine, Institute for Women's Health,
                         University College London Hospitals, UK

Karen Racicot   Assistant Professor, Department of Obstetrics,
                         Gynecology and Reproductive Biology,
                         College of Human Medicine, Michigan State
                         University, USA

Raymond W Redline   Professor of Pathology, Case Western Reserve
                         University; University Hospitals Case Medical
                         Center, Ohio, USA

Colin Sibley   Professor of Child Health and Physiology,
                         Maternal and Fetal Health Research Centre,
                         Institute of Human Development, University of
                         Manchester, UK

Philip Steer   Emeritus Professor of Obstetrics and
                         Gynaecology, Imperial College London, UK

Suresh Victor   Senior Attending Physician, Neonatology
                         Center of Excellence, Sidra Medical and
                         Research Center, Doha, Qatar

Michael Weindling   Emeritus Professor of Perinatal Medicine,
                         Department of Women's and Children's
                         Health, University of Liverpool, UK

Melissa Westwood   Professor of Endocrinology, Maternal and Fetal
                         Health Research Centre, Institute of Human
                         Development, University of Manchester, UK

FOREWORD

The development of the human brain in fetal life is of critical importance for lifelong function. Many neurodevelopmental deficits originate in the perinatal period and there is increasing awareness of the need to look into early life, including prenatal life, to understand the origins of cognitive development, healthy ageing and risk of neurodegenerative and psychiatric diseases.

The first edition of this book, edited by Philip Baker and Colin Sibley and published in 2006, drew attention to the role of utero-placental function as an important mediator of healthy fetal brain development. Since then there have been significant advances in this topic from a range of disciplines, including epidemiology, histopathology, endocrinology, imaging science, immunology, neuroprotection studies and rigorous assessment of clinical outcomes. Consequently, publication of a second edition that encompasses the new breadth of understanding is important and timely. This book succeeds unequivocally in addressing this need.

The book is structured in a logical way from pathology to clinical outcome. Throughout, information from the basic sciences is placed within the clinical context and there is excellent use of illustrative figures and images. These aspects of design and structure ensure that the volume is readily accessible to a broad readership.

All of the chapters are valuable. Redline's chapter on placental pathology and perinatal brain injury sets the tone superbly and Sibley and Desforges continue to provide a detailed unifying theory of aberrant placentation and development, offering explanations for inadequate placental function and fetal compromise. The chapters by Charnock and Westwood, Crocker, and Racicot and Mor consider the roles of endocrine systems, placental haemodynamics and inflammation respectively, in placentation and function. There follows an excellent contribution from Peebles and James on infection and the fetal inflammatory response. Victor and Weindling discuss the synergy between inflammation and hypoxia-ischaemia as mediators of white matter injury and Cetin and Brusati discuss the problem of disturbed cerebral energetics in fetal growth restriction. There follow chapters on state-of-the-art methods for assessing placental structure, function and perfusion as well as fetal well-being using magnetic resonance imaging and ultrasound (Ingram and Johnstone), and magnetic resonance spectroscopy (Cetin and Brusati). Abel and Allin present the compelling case for the importance of prenatal factors on the causal pathway to psychiatric disease, while Steer provides a thorough overview of current strategies for fetal neuroprotection. Dr Nelson's summary and discussion of knowledge gaps about the role of the placenta in fetal brain development provide an elegant and thought-provoking final chapter to this volume.

The editors should be congratulated for bringing together a panel of expert authors from diverse fields and for editing a volume that is comprehensive and authoritative. It should prove to be a valuable resource for basic scientists, obstetricians, neonatologists and pathologists and all those engaged in understanding the complex interactions between placental function and fetal brain development, as a basis for improving health outcomes across the life-course.

Dr James P Boardman
MRC Centre for Reproductive Health
University of Edinburgh
UK

PREFACE

The original concept and first edition of this book on placenta and neurodisability was developed from a meeting organised by Martin Bax and Mac Keith Meetings, held in the UK almost a decade ago with the support of the Castang Foundation. Over the intervening years, the links between this unique organ and the human brain, in utero as well as beyond, have expanded, aided not least by the continued enthusiasm and evangelism of Dr Bax and like-minded individuals. With a second meeting in 2010, it became obvious that knowledge, understanding and certainty in this topic had progressed, alongside clinical and technical advances and that a reworking of the original volume was necessary and somewhat overdue. Many participants at this meeting have contributed to this new edition and thankfully have formalised their links to expedite clinical and research progress across international borders.

As highlighted, neurodisability relating to perinatal brain injury is recognised in 2 to 3 of every 1000 live births. However, the numbers associated with more subtle, late-onset neurophysical disorders, perhaps exacerbated by environmental factors, may be more profound. As is evident throughout the text, improvements in obstetric care and neonatal surveillance have served to increase infant survival, particularly for those of very low birthweight and defined contributory lesions. Nevertheless, iatrogenic stresses remain a concern, with overriding importance given to developmental immaturity, underlying fetal growth restriction, cardiopulmonary instability and infections, placental or otherwise. In many cases, placental pathology provides a circumscribed role, identifying inflammatory responses and functional deficits. Nevertheless, for cases of neurodisability at term or in the near-term infant, it is becoming increasingly clear, as indicated in this book, that the placenta has a major role in the pathophysiology which underscores, or at the very least contributes, to central nervous system injury and dysplasia.

To this end, this book covers all necessary components and discussion points regarding these placental contributions, from inflammation (infectious and immunological) through aberrations in placental and fetal growth, the role of genetic and environmental factors in neurological development, along with current clinical approaches to monitoring and restricting aberrations. Nevertheless, as emphasised by Karin Nelson in the final chapter, more work lies ahead. Along with clarification of the fetal-placental insults which beget developmental issues, there is a specific need for follow-up studies in humans to delineate disorders, strenghthen associations with placental pathophysiology and define the biological foundations of congenital neurodisability. Only when these are determined will progress in preventing and offsetting this string of pathological events be forthcoming, with a possible leap forward in fetal and perinatal medicine. Nonetheless, as a marker of current knowledge in all aspects of this complex story, this book stands alone in its breadth and accessibility, to be read by experts and inquisitive minds alike.

Ian Crocker
Maternal and Fetal Health Research Centre
University of Manchester, UK
April 2015

1

PLACENTAL PATHOLOGY IN UNDERSTANDING PERINATAL BRAIN INJURY

Raymond W Redline

Introduction

Static disorders of motor function, such as cerebral palsy (CP), develop within the first two years of life in approximately 2 – 3/1000 children (Himmelmann et al. 2010). Depending on the regional prevalence of premature birth (especially at less than 28 weeks gestation), the proportion of cases related to extreme immaturity may vary from between 25 and 50%. In almost all cohorts the proportion of otherwise unremarkable term infants (> 37 wks) is relatively constant at around 40% – 50%. The remaining cases are a heterogeneous group, including near term infants, markedly growth restricted infants of all gestational ages, infants with undiagnosed genetic or chromosomal disorders and infants with neurotoxic exposures to infectious agents or other toxins in either the prenatal or postnatal period.

Recognized clinical risk factors for CP and related disorders in the extremely preterm infant include earlier gestational age, superimposed fetal growth restriction, a low Apgar score at birth, postnatal hypoxia, overly aggressive ventilation with hyperoxia–hypocarbia, patent ductus arteriosus, postnatal corticosteroid therapy and postnatal inflammatory disorders including necrotizing enterocolitis and late onset sepsis (Babcock et al. 2009). The degree of risk associated with ascending bacterial infections (chorioamnionitis), as discussed below, remains controversial and is considered in Chapter 6. Recognized risk factors for central nervous system (CNS) injury in term infants include a positive family history of neurodevelopmental disorders, fetal growth restriction, abnormal neurological examination in the first days of life (neonatal encephalopathy) and hypothyroidism (Redline 2008a). The degree of risk associated with so-called birth asphyxia (recently defined by several international consensus conferences) is also controversial and will be discussed later in the book. Novel therapies decreasing the susceptibility of neurons to injury, including magnesium sulfate in preterm infants and head cooling in term infants, raise the possibility of attenuating CNS injury associated with acute insults, but may be less efficacious in cases with coexisting placental pathology.

The existing literature on placental pathology and CNS injury suffers from several problems. First, adverse outcomes are rare and often diagnosed years after birth. Other limitations include bias of ascertainment, lack of an appropriate control group, inadequate characterization of placental lesions, use of surrogate short-term outcomes, unmeasurable differences in genetic susceptibility to injury and failure to fully account for the effects of gestational age and post birth complications. Nevertheless, contrary to the conclusions of a recent commentary (Nelson and Blair 2011), strong working hypotheses have emerged from the large number of published reports regarding which types of placental lesions are most likely to increase the risk of CNS injury. The focus of this chapter will be to place these pathologic findings in perspective in terms of their ability to cause or alter the threshold for the various manifestations of perinatal brain injury including abnormal neuroimaging, neonatal encephalopathy, ischemic stroke, seizure disorders and later disabilities such as CP and developmental delay in live born infants and neuropathological changes in stillbirths.

Potential placental mechanisms for injury
The placenta is essential for fetal life; constituting its only source for oxygen, water, nutrients and elimination of waste products. So in a sense it is not surprising that placental dysfunction can lead to disordered growth and development or injury to specific organs such as the brain and spinal cord. However, it has been challenging to isolate the particular patterns of placental injury that are most likely to cause damage. Before considering specific placental lesions, the potential pathways by which placental dysfunction could affect fetal brain function will be briefly reviewed.

PAUCITY OF PROTECION
In this scenario the fetus is deprived of specific crucial elements such as essential amino acids, maternal or placental hormones, or minerals and vitamins that are necessary for CNS development or protection from injury (Dammann and Leviton 1999). One simple way this can occur is preterm birth, that is, severing the fetus from its maternal supply line. Other potential mechanisms include genetic or epigenetic abnormalities in placental transporters or growth factor expression and maternal deficiencies in dietary intake or metabolic state. While these pathways may be extremely important, as evidenced by the importance of a positive family history and the known effects of maternal hypothyroidism and phenylketonuria on later childhood CNS function, they have no known structural correlate and cannot be detected by pathological examination.

DYSFUNCTION OF CORE PATHWAYS
The supply line between mother and fetus depends on adequate maternal circulating volume and blood pressure; an intact and appropriately remodeled utero-placental vasculature; free circulation through and drainage of the placental intervillous spaces; a short diffusion distance between maternal blood and fetal capillaries; and an intact, non-obstructed feto-placental circulation (see Fig. 1.1). Pathophysiological processes directly affecting these core pathways fall into two categories. The first category includes acute sentinel events such as maternal shock, uterine rupture, abruptio placenta, umbilical cord occlusion and feto-placental hemorrhages. These often result in either fetal death or recovery without CNS sequelae, but in some cases lead to global asphyxia and later CP with major developmental disabilities (Myers 1975). The second category includes chronic sub-lethal processes

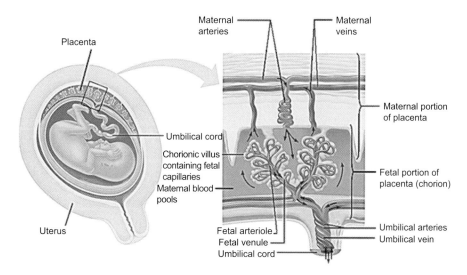

Fig. 1.1. Topological depiction of the human placenta, showing main structural elements and maternal and fetal blood flow. Reproduced by permission Pearson Education © 2013.

leading to gradual loss of function and decreased placental reserve to withstand later injury (i.e. situations where fetal demand exceeds placental supply). Processes associated with decreased placental reserve include maternal malperfusion (MMP), secondary to inadequate maternal vascular remodeling, inadequate placental mass (placental weight less than 10th centile for gestational age) and processes affecting the diffusing capacity across the interhemal membrane (placental maturation defect, perivillous fibrin(oid) deposition and villitis of unknown etiology [VUE]), that is unexplained villus infiltration by maternal T lymphocytes.

DISTURBANCES INVOLVING MULTIPLE DISTINCT PHYSIOLOIC COMPARTMENTS
Numerous studies have shown that CNS injury is strongly associated with multiple placental lesions (so-called 'mixed pathology'). These lesions may act synergistically to disrupt a single core pathway or in parallel by blocking both primary and compensatory pathways. They can act either directly by affecting gas exchange or indirectly via the elaboration of harmful circulating mediators including cytokines, pathogen or damage associated molecular patterns (PAMP/DAMP), complement fragments, microparticles, activated coagulation components, vasoactive molecules and reactive oxygen species. It is important to distinguish the finding of multiple independent lesions from multiple abnormalities that all characterize a single pattern of injury (so-called constellation disorders).

PRECONDITIONING INVOLVING PLACENTAL LESIONS OCCURING AT DIFFEREENT TIMES
The general hypothesis of preconditioning is that changes of state induced by prior events can either positively or negatively modulate the deleterious effects of a subsequent insult

(Hagberg et al. 2004). In the placenta these sequential insults generally involve repeated exposure to hypoxia, circulating inflammatory mediators, or some combination of the two. However, they could also potentially include placental conditions that alter the fetal endocrine or metabolic state. The concept of preconditioning helps to explain the inconsistent association of any single placental lesion with CNS injury. Since preconditioning can also be positive, this may explain why in some studies processes such as chorioamnionitis and mild MMP have actually been found to be neuroprotective.

Placental pathology in CNS injury
Key characteristics of a good pathological study include the use of clearly defined and generally accepted findings that characterize interruption of a specific physiological pathway, incorporation of scaling that distinguishes the intensity (grade), duration (stage), extent and character of these findings and comparison with an appropriate control group. Ideally specific criteria for each finding should be fully described as reproducibility of these findings is an important consideration for clinical application and studies involving multiple different scorers. However this is not a central issue for studies undertaken in a single center or where scoring is done at a central reading center. Unfortunately, few studies have met all of these benchmarks. This, combined, with the logistic issues and clinical confounders mentioned above, contributes to continuing skepticism regarding the validity of placental pathology in helping to explain adverse neurological outcomes.

PATTERNS ASSOCIATED WITH CNS INJURY AT ALL GESTATIONAL AGES
Several types of placental injury have been consistently associated with different types of CNS injury in diverse clinical scenarios at all gestational ages. The identification of more than one placental lesion has been the strongest and most consistent predictor between studies and is the finding least influenced by other risk factors and confounders (Redline and O'Riordan 2000, Viscardi and Sun 2001, Chang et al. 2011). Also, the degree of risk has been shown to increase significantly with each additional placental lesion identified. The most commonly observed combinations are a vascular lesion (either maternal or fetal) with an inflammatory process (either acute or chronic); however combinations of a maternal and fetal vascular lesion or acute and chronic inflammation are also seen.

A second set of findings in diverse types of CNS injury are placental changes indicative of severe MMP, such as villous infarction (Fig. 1.2a). These have been associated with neuronal necrosis in stillborn fetuses, CP and developmental delay in preterm infants and CP in association with neonatal encephalopathy in term infants (Burke and Tannenberg 1995, Redline et al. 2007). A much less common form of maternal perfusion abnormality known as maternal floor infarction has also been associated with both motor disorders and developmental delay at all gestational ages (Adams-Chapman et al. 2002).

Finally, pathological findings suggestive of chronic partial or intermittent umbilical cord obstruction, have also been implicated in several studies of CNS injury (Grafe 1994, Redline 2008b). The biological plausibility for this pattern is supported by neurological follow-up in infants with sonographic evidence of persistent cord entanglements and animal

4

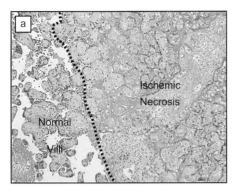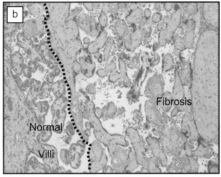

Fig. 1.2. Placental vascular lesions with high prevalence in neonatal brain injury. (a) Maternal villous infarct: A portion of the distal villous tree shows ischemic necrosis of villous trophoblast and obliteration of the intervillous space, secondary to obstruction of a maternal spiral artery. Villous stromal and vascular architecture is preserved. Normal villi are seen on the left (H&E stain, 10x magnification). (b) Fetal thrombotic vasculopathy: A portion of the distal villous tree shows loss of fetal vessels and stromal fibrosis secondary to obstruction of a large fetal placental vessel. Villous trophoblast and intervillous space are preserved. Normal villi seen on the left side (H&E stain, 10x magnification). A colour version of this figure can be seen in the plate section at the end of the book.

studies documenting the effects of repetitive episodes of fetal hypoxia and partial prolonged asphyxia (Myers 1975, Clapp et al. 2003). Gross pathological lesions affecting the umbilical cord, such as membranous insertion, excessive length, increased coiling and tight knots can all potentially restrict feto-placental blood flow. When combined with histological indicators, such as scattered small foci of avascular villi, intimal fibrin cushions in stem villous vessels, perivascular edema around stem villous arteries, distal villous immaturity and chorionic/stem villous venous dilation at the cord insertion site, they can cause a physiologically significant reduction in umbilical blood flow, increased placental venous pressure and fetal vascular stasis.

PATTERNS ASSOCIATED WITH CNS INJURY IN PRETERM INFANTS

The majority of studies addressing CNS injury in preterm infants have focused on histologic chorioamnionitis (HCA). Although meta-analysis has found HCA to be a significant risk factor for CP, the exact nature of the relationship remains unclear (Shatrov et al. 2010). Several specific problems confound this association: (1) the prevalence of HCA increases dramatically with decreasing gestational age, the strongest predictor of CNS injury in this population; (2) HCA is highly prevalent in this population (over 50%) and often seen with precipitous uncontrolled vaginal deliveries, while other less frequent causes of preterm birth (twins, pre-eclampsia) are often more closely monitored and more likely to undergo elective operative deliveries; (3) HCA-negative comparison groups are enriched for placentas with mild MMP, which may exert a protective effect against CNS injury (see below); (4) HCA predisposes to post-birth neonatal complications that may themselves be the cause of injury; and (5) HCA is a complex mixture of different grades and stages of maternal and fetal inflammation that have not been adequately separated in many studies.

In placentas with HCA the strongest and most consistent risk factor for CNS injury is acute fetal vasculitis affecting either umbilical (funisitis) or chorionic plate (chorionic vasculitis) vessels. Fetal vasculitis is not a true vasculitis, but rather transmigration of fetally-derived neutrophils toward bacteria in the amniotic fluid. When found in umbilical arteries, compared with the umbilical vein alone, fetal vasculitis has been correlated with elevated levels of fetal cytokines (Rogers et al. 2002). Specific outcomes in preterm infants that have been associated with HCA with or without FV include intraventricular hemorrhage, white matter lesions on early head ultrasound and developmental delay at various periods during childhood (Leviton et al. 1999, Mittendorf et al. 2003). Other studies have shown that increased intensity of FV, recent non-occlusive fetal thrombi and maternal perfusion abnormalities all increase the risk of injury with HCA (Redline et al 1998, Kaukola et al. 2006). However, a few studies have found that HCA is associated with a decreased risk of death and no change in the risk of neurological impairment, illustrating the continuing controversy regarding the exact nature of this relationship (Dexter et al. 2000, Andrews et al. 2008).

Additional placental lesions that have been associated with more than one pattern of CNS injury in preterm infants include diffuse villous edema, severe MMP and two decidual lesions, recent hemorrhage and fibrin and lymphoplasmacytic inflammation (Kumazaki et al. 2002, Mehta et al. 2006, Redline et al. 2007, Maleki et al. 2009, Leviton et al. 2010). Interestingly, mild MMP was associated with a reduced risk of adverse outcomes in one study (Redline et al. 1998).

Patterns associated with CNS injury in term infants

Methodological issues such as the inability to identify infants at risk and a lack of appropriate controls, have made the study of placental pathology and CNS injury in term infants particularly difficult. Observations in specific cohorts such as cases in litigation, infants with neonatal encephalopathy, tertiary care referrals for head cooling and stillbirths with detailed neuropathologic examination provide some insight. Fetal thrombotic vasculopathy (FTV, Fig. 1.2b) and other pathological processes damaging large feto-placental vessels in the umbilical cord and/or chorionic plate (VUE with obliterative fetal vasculopathy, meconium-associated fetal vascular necrosis and HCA with intense fetal vasculitis) have emerged as highly prevalent and strongly significant predictors of CNS injury. In the largest studies, these have been specifically associated with neuronal damage, neonatal encephalopathy and CP (McDonald et al. 2004, Redline 2005, Chang et al. 2011). Although often seen in cases of intrapartum distress, their effects appear to be independent of indicators of birth asphyxia such as low cord pH and 5 minute Apgar score. In term infants referred for head cooling they have been found by some, but not all, investigators to predict a decreased responsiveness to therapy compared with infants showing evidence of birth asphyxia alone (Wintermark et al. 2010, Ernst et al. 2012).

Other pathologic lesions associated with CNS injury in term placentas include heterochronic placental lesions (one present for weeks, the other present for 6 – 12 hours or more), scattered foci of avascular villi suggestive of umbilical cord obstruction and placental infarcts (Redline and O'Riordan 2000, Redline 2008, Nelson and Blair 2011).

In smaller studies, placental maturation defect and FTV were found to be more prevalent in children with perinatal stroke, whilst placental maturation defect and VUE were more prevalent in infants with seizures (Scher et al. 1998, Elbers et al. 2011).

Pathological approach
Finally, leaving theoretical and epidemiological considerations aside, I will briefly describe how I, as a pathologist and medico-legal consultant, approach the relationship between specific placental lesions and CNS injury in individual cases. I generally subdivide cases into six categories. These categories are hierarchical in the sense that earlier categories take precedence over later ones. However, the finding of lesions in multiple categories is very common and undoubtedly increases the risk of significant CNS damage.

1: LESIONS SUFFICIENT ALONE TO EXPLAIN CNS INJURY
These are the so-called 'sentinel events' such as abruptio placenta, uterine rupture, fetal hemorrhage, or complete umbilical cord obstruction. Since these lesions cause critical hypoxia they are almost by definition acute, occurring within a period of minutes to hours before birth. Placental findings consistent with sentinel events are generally identified at gross examination and include large retroplacental hematomas, torn fetal vessels, or tight umbilical cord knots. Microscopic examination is generally supplementary to the clinical history and gross examination in these situations. Placental evaluation can sometimes change the clinical diagnosis of a sentinel event by failing to substantiate the clinical impression and/or by identifying alternative explanations.

2: LESIONS SUFFICIENT ALONE TO EXPLAIN CNS INJURY, BUT USUALLY SEEN IN COMBINATION WITH
   INTRAPARTUM DISTRESS
The main diagnoses in this category are the thrombotic and inflammatory lesions that affect large fetal placental blood vessels including FTV, VUE with obliterative fetal vasculopathy and prolonged meconium exposure with vascular necrosis. Another inflammatory lesion, chorioamnionitis with an intense fetal vasculitis, has been reported as a risk factor in some studies, particularly when combined with recent non-occlusive chorionic vessel thrombi in preterm infants. These types of lesions not only affect placental function, but can also compromise fetal circulatory physiology and directly cause fetal organ damage via the effects of circulating mediators such as cytokines, microparticles and activated coagulation components.

3: LESIONS SUFFICIENT TO CAUSE INJURY, BUT OF LOWER SPECIFICITY
These lesions are also highly prevalent in cases of CNS injury, but overlap with findings observed in placentas submitted for other reasons. Three lesions in this category are chronic partial/intermittent umbilical cord obstruction, marked MMP and diffuse villous edema. The first two are so-called 'constellation disorders' that depend on the identification of multiple related findings. In these processes it can be difficult to decide which combinations of findings are most specific for significant placental dysfunction. Further studies are needed to dissect patterns and severities that allow more accurate prediction. One finding

that can assist in assessing the degree of associated hypoxia is an elevation in the number of immature red blood cell precursors in the fetal placental circulation (see below). The third lesion in this category, diffuse villous edema, is only seen in the placentas of extremely low gestational age preterm infants. There is some ambiguity related to this lesion since it is somewhat subjective and an exaggeration of a normal developmental pattern seen in late second trimester placentas. Nevertheless, it has been a strong predictor across studies and is independent of gestational age by multivariate analysis.

4: Lesions usually not sufficient alone to cause injury, but synergistic with intrapartum stress

Lesions in this category decrease the placental reserve by compromising the efficiency of placental function. While not directly causal, they can decrease the threshold for comparatively minor episodes of perinatal stress to compromise CNS function. Most cases of MMP, distal villous immaturity/placental maturation defect, VUE without obliterative vasculopathy, chronic abruption and perivillous fibrinoid deposition without maternal floor infarction fall within this category.

5: Non-causal adaptive lesions indicative of antenatal stress

There are two lesions in this category: villous chorangiosis and increased circulating fetal nucleated red blood cells (NRBC). Chorangiosis reflects increased villous angiogenesis developing over weeks in response to decreased maternal oxygen tension with normal maternal perfusion. Recognized associations include maternal anemia, smoking and pregnancy at high altitudes (Ogino and Redline 2000). Significantly increased circulating NRBC (more than one per high power field, corresponding to a neonatal count of greater than 2500/mm3) represent a physiologic response to decreased fetal oxygen tension with mobilization of immature red blood cell precursors from intramedullary and extramedullary sources (Redline 2008b). Significantly elevated NRBC counts are believed to develop after a period of at least 6–12 hours of significant tissue hypoxia.

6. No identifiable placental lesion

This final category is heterogeneous. Explanations to consider when placentas show no significant lesions include unrecognized clinical sentinel events, birth trauma, inadequate placental examination and intrinsic CNS susceptibility due to genetic or epigenetic abnormalities. The latter explanation is most plausible when a positive family history of neurodevelopmental disorders exists.

Conclusions

Extrinsic factors aside, a unifying hypothesis to account for the relationship between the placenta and CNS injury is that, between 23 and 39 weeks' gestation there exists a critical period for brain development and resilience to injury that requires a fully functioning placenta. Birth before this stage (paucity of protection) and placental dysfunction during this stage (decreased reserve and preconditioning) can decrease the threshold for problems in the perinatal period. These placental processes also interact with inherent variations in the set point for CNS injury, a variable that is likely to be influenced by poorly understood genetic and epigenetic factors. Together with better understanding of relevant physiology and genetics and better epidemiological studies, the development of antenatal screening tests to identify fetuses and placentas at risk is a major goal for the prevention, early diagnosis and prompt treatment of perinatal brain damage.

REFERENCES

Adams-Chapman I, Vaucher YE, Bejar RF, Benirschke K, Baergen RN, Moore TR (2002) Maternal floor infarction of the placenta: Association with central nervous system injury and adverse neurodevelopmental outcome. *J Perinatol* 22(3): 236–241. doi: http://dx.doi.org/10.1038/sj.jp.7210685

Andrews WW, Cliver SP, Biasini F et al. (2008) Early preterm birth: Association between in utero exposure to acute inflammation and severe neurodevelopmental disability at 6 years of age. *Am J Obstet Gynecol* 198(4): 466.e1–466.e11. doi: http://dx.doi.org/10.1016/j.ajog.2007.12.031

Babcock MA, Kostova FV, Ferriero DM et al. (2009) Injury to the preterm brain and cerebral palsy: Clinical aspects, molecular mechanisms, unanswered questions, and future research directions. *J Child Neurol* 24(9): 1064–1084. doi: http://dx.doi.org/10.1177/0883073809338957

Blair E, de Groot J, Nelson KB (2011) Placental infarction identified by macroscopic examination and risk of cerebral palsy in infants at 35 weeks of gestational age and over. *Am J Obstet Gynecol* 205(2): 124. e1–124.e7. doi: http://dx.doi.org/10.1016/j.ajog.2011.05.022

Burke CJ, Tannenberg AE (1995) Prenatal brain damage and placental infarction: An autopsy study. *Dev Med Child Neurol* 37: 555–562. doi: http://dx.doi.org/10.1111/j.1469-8749.1995.tb12042.x

Chang KT, Keating S, Costa S, Machin G, Kingdom J, Shannon P (2011) Third-trimester stillbirths: Correlative neuropathology and placental pathology. *Pediatr Dev Pathol* 14(5): 345–352. doi: http://dx.doi.org/10.2350/10-07-0882-oa.1

Clapp JF III, Stepanchak W, Hashimoto K, Ehrenberg H, Lopez B (2003) The natural history of antenatal nuchal cords. *Am J Obstet Gynecol* 189(2): 488–493. doi: http://dx.doi.org/10.1067/s0002-9378(03)00371-5

Dammann O, Leviton A (1999) Brain damage in preterm newborns: Might enhancement of developmentally regulated endogenous protection open a door for prevention? *Pediatrics* 104(3 Pt 1): 541–550.

Dexter SC, Pinar H, Malee MP, Hogan J, Carpenter MW, Vohr BR (2000) Outcome of very low birth weight infants with histopathologic chorioamnionitis. *Obstet Gynecol* 96(2): 172–177. doi: http://dx.doi.org/10.1016/s0029-7844(00)00886-3

Elbers J, Viero S, MacGregor D, deVeber G, Moore AM (2011) Placental pathology in neonatal stroke. *Pediatrics* 127(3): e722–e729. doi: http://dx.doi.org/10.1542/peds.2010-1490

Ernst LM, de Regnier RO, Boswell L, Huang MH, Khan JY (2012) Clinicopathologic factors as predictors of outcome in term infants with hypoxic ischemic encephalopathy undergoing therapeutic hypothermia. *Pediatr Dev Pathol* 14: 510–511.

Grafe MR (1994) The correlation of prenatal brain damage with placental pathology. *Neuropathol Exp Neurol* 53: 407–415. doi: http://dx.doi.org/10.1097/00005072-199407000-00013

Hagberg H, Dammann O, Mallard C, Leviton A (2004) Preconditioning and the developing brain. *Semin Perinatol* 28(6): 389–395. doi: http://dx.doi.org/10.1053/j.semperi.2004.10.006

Himmelmann K, Hagberg G, Uvebrant P (2010) The changing panorama of cerebral palsy in Sweden. X. Prevalence and origin in the birth-year period 1999–2002. *Acta Paediatr* 99(9): 1337–1343. doi: http://dx.doi.org/10.1111/j.1651-2227.2010.01819.x

Kaukola T, Herva R, Perhomaa M et al. (2006). Population cohort associating chorioamnionitis, cord inflammatory cytokines and neurologic outcome in very preterm, extremely low birth weight infants. *Pediatr Res* 59(3): 478–483. doi: http://dx.doi.org/10.1203/01.pdr.0000182596.66175.ee

Kumazaki K, Nakayama M, Sumida Y et al. (2002). Placental features in preterm infants with periventricular leukomalacia. *Pediatrics* 109(4): 650–655. doi: http://dx.doi.org/10.1542/peds.109.4.650

Leviton A, Allred EN, Kuban KCK et al. (2010) Microbiologic and histologic characteristics of the extremely preterm infant's placenta predict white matter damage and later cerebral palsy. The ELGAN study. *Pediatr Res* 67(1): 95–101. doi: http://dx.doi.org/10.1203/pdr.0b013e3181bf5fab

Leviton A, Paneth N, Lynne Reuss M et al. (1999) Maternal infection, fetal inflammatory response and brain damage in very low birth weight infants. Developmental Epidemiology Network Investigators. *Pediatr Res* 46(5): 566–575. doi: http://dx.doi.org/10.1203/00006450-199911000-00013

Maleki Z, Bailis AJ, Argani CH, Askin FB, Graham EM (2009). Periventricular leukomalacia and placental histopathologic abnormalities. *Obstet Gynecol* 114(5): 1115–1120. doi: http://dx.doi.org/10.1097/aog.0b013e3181bdcfc4

McDonald DG, Kelehan P, McMenamin JB et al. (2004). Placental fetal thrombotic vasculopathy is associated with neonatal encephalopathy. *Hum Pathol* 35(7): 875–880. doi: http://dx.doi.org/10.1016/j.humpath.2004.02.014

Mehta R, Nanjundaswamy S, Shen-Schwarz S, Petrova A (2006). Neonatal morbidity and placental pathology. *Indian J Pediatr* 73(1): 25–28. doi: http://dx.doi.org/10.1007/bf02758255

Mittendorf R, Montag AG, MacMillan W et al. (2003). Components of the systemic fetal inflammatory response syndrome as predictors of impaired neurologic outcomes in children. *Am J Obstet Gynecol* 188(6): 1438–1446. doi: http://dx.doi.org/10.1067/mob.2003.380

Myers RE (1975) Four patterns of perinatal brain damage and their conditions of occurrence in primates. *Adv Neurol* 10: 223–234.

Nelson KB, Blair E (2011) The placenta and neurologic and psychiatric outcomes in the child: Study design matters. *Placenta* 32(9): 623–625. doi: http://dx.doi.org/10.1016/j.placenta.2011.06.021

Ogino S, Redline RW (2000) Villous capillary lesions of the placenta: Distinctions between chorangioma, chorangiomatosis and chorangiosis. *Hum Pathol* 31: 945–954. doi: http://dx.doi.org/10.1053/hupa.2000.9036

Redline RW (2005) Severe fetal placental vascular lesions in term infants with neurologic impairment. *Am J Obstet Gynecol* 192: 452–457. doi: http://dx.doi.org/10.1016/j.ajog.2004.07.030

Redline RW (2008a) Cerebral palsy in term infants: A clinicopathologic analysis of 158 medicolegal case reviews. *Pediatr Dev Pathol* 11(6): 456–464. doi: http://dx.doi.org/10.2350/08-05-0468.1

Redline RW (2008b) Elevated circulating fetal nucleated red blood cells and placental pathology in term infants who develop cerebral palsy. *Hum Pathol* 39(9): 1378–1384. doi: http://dx.doi.org/10.1016/j.humpath.2008.01.017

Redline RW, Minich N, Gerry Taylor H, Hack M (2007). Placental lesions as predictors of cerebral palsy and abnormal neurocognitive function at school age in extremely low birth weight infants (<1 kg). *Pediatr Dev Pathol* 10(4): 282–292. doi: http://dx.doi.org/10.2350/06-12-0203.1

Redline RW, O'Riordan MA (2000) Placental lesions associated with cerebral palsy and neurologic impairment following term birth. *Arch Pathol Lab Med* 124(12): 1785–1791.

Redline RW, Wilson-Costello D, Borawski E, Fanaroff AA, Hack M (1998). Placental lesions associated with neurologic impairment and cerebral palsy in very low birth weight infants. *Arch Pathol Lab Med* 122: 1091–1098.

Rogers BB, Alexander JM, Head J, Mcintire D, Leveno KJ (2002) Umbilical vein interleukin-6 levels correlate with the severity of placental inflammation and gestational age. *Hum Pathol* 33(3): 335–340. doi: http://dx.doi.org/10.1053/hupa.2002.32214

Scher MS, Trucco GS, Beggarly ME, Steppe DA, Macpherson TA (1998) Neonates with electrically confirmed seizures and possible placental associations. *Pediatr Neurol* 19: 37–41. doi: http://dx.doi.org/10.1016/s0887-8994(98)00012-5

Shatrov JG, Birch SC, Lam LT, Quinlivan JA, McIntyre S, Mendz GL (2010). Chorioamnionitis and cerebral palsy: A meta-analysis. *Obstet Gynecol* 116(2 Pt 1): 387–392. doi: http://dx.doi.org/10.1097/aog.0b013e3181e90046

Viscardi RM, Sun CC (2001). Placental lesion multiplicity: Risk factor for IUGR and neonatal cranial ultrasound abnormalities. *Early Hum Dev* 62(1): 1–10. doi: http://dx.doi.org/10.1016/s0378-3782(01)00114-1

Wintermark P, Boyd T, Gregas MC, Labrecque M, Hansen A (2010). Placental pathology in asphyxiated newborns meeting the criteria for therapeutic hypothermia. *Am J Obstet Gynecol* 203(6): 579.e1–579.e9. doi: http://dx.doi.org/10.1016/j.ajog.2010.08.024

2
ABNORMAL PLACENTAL PHENOTYPES

Colin Sibley and Michelle Desforges

Over the last 60 years, advancing knowledge has allowed us to progress from a situation where the placenta was considered a simple sieve between maternal and fetal blood (Flexner and Gellhorn, 1942) to our current understanding of the placenta as a key mediator and regulator of maternal supply and fetal demand for nutrients necessary for growth and organogenesis (Reik et al., 2003). It is now clear that abnormal placental structure and morphology, together with placental dysfunction and ultimately failure, have a causal role in major pregnancy diseases, such as fetal growth restriction (FGR) and preterm birth, pregnancy issues with pronounced neurodevelopmental implications (Baschat, 2011). The accurate diagnosis of pregnancies at risk remains improbable. However, with growing understanding of placental function, in normal and complicated pregnancies, the placenta is now taking centre-stage as a focus for this diagnosis. Here we detail how placental phenotyping may aid the clinician in identifying at-risk infants, using the abnormal placental phenotypes associated with FGR as exemplar.

Placental phenotyping in fetal growth restriction: placental transport
By definition, when a fetus is growth restricted, there has been less net transfer of nutrients across the placenta. The question arises as to what determinants of transfer capacity have been altered. Ultimately the capacity of the placenta to transfer nutrients and waste is dependent on (1) placental structure and function and (2) maternal and/or fetal environments. The main determinants of placental nutrient transfer are discussed below, with reference to normal pregnancy and FGR. For guidance, Figure 2.1 depicts the normal exchange barrier of the human placenta and Figure 2.2 summarises the mechanisms of placental exchange.

Transfer gradients: normal pregnancy
Concentration, electrical and hydrostatic gradients between maternal and fetal plasma across the placental exchange barrier (depicted in Fig. 2.1) provide the driving force for transfer. The concentration gradient of any solute will affect its rate of transfer via any mechanism (see diffusion and transporter-mediated processes below). Maternal plasma solute concentrations will be dependent on maternal homeostasis, including the rate at which the placenta transfers or absorbs particular solutes; fetal plasma concentrations will also be dependent on placental transfer as well as fetal metabolic processes.

Electrical gradients will affect the transfer by diffusion of charged solutes such as ions or the cationic and anionic amino acids. The magnitude and polarity of the electrical gradient, or potential difference across the placental exchange barrier is still uncertain, though

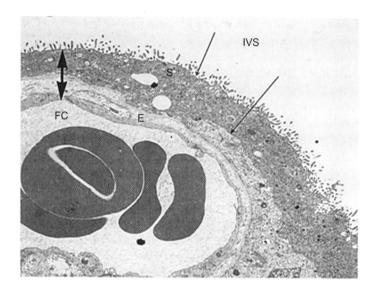

Fig. 2.1. Electron micrograph image (courtesy of CJP Jones) of the placental exchange barrier. Single-headed arrows identify the microvillous (maternal facing) and basal (fetal facing) plasma membranes of the syncytiotrophoblast. Double-headed arrow demonstrates entire barrier, across which transfer between maternal and fetal blood takes place. Reproduced from *Int J Dev Biol* (2010) 54: 377–390 with permission from University of the Basque Country Press. IVS, intervillous space containing maternal blood; FC, fetal capillary containing fetal blood; S, syncytiotrophoblast; E, fetal capillary endothelium.

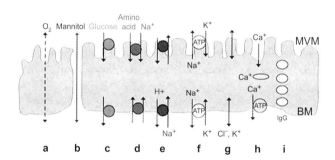

Fig. 2.2. Schematic diagram of the major mechanisms of transfer across the placental microvillous membrane (MVM) and basal membrane (BPM) of the syncytiotrophoblast: (a) simple diffusion of relatively lipophilic substances; (b) paracellular route for hydrophilic substances: (c–h) transporter-mediated transport: (c) facilitated diffusion; (d) co-transport; (e) exchange; and (f,h) active transport. ATP; adenosine triphosphate. Ion channels (g,h) are present in the MVM and BPM and there is evidence for endocytosis–exocytosis (i). Examples of solutes transported by each mechanism are included. Reproduced from *Int J Dev Biol* (2010) 54: 377–390 with permission from University of the Basque Country Press. A colour version of this figure can be seen in the plate section at the end of the book.

in vitro it is about 6 mV, fetal side negative (Greenwood et al. 1993). Theoretically, this may be generated through maternal and fetal homeostasis creating a concentration gradient in charged solute or through active transport by the placenta of these solutes (e.g. Na^+ transfer utilising the Na^+/K^+ ATPase; see Fig. 2.2).

Hydrostatic pressure gradients will drive transfer of water by bulk flow. The pressures in the intervillous space on the maternal side of the placental exchange barrier and in the fetal capillaries on the other side will be determined by cardiac output from the respective hearts and resistance in the vascular trees. These pressures in the intervillous space and fetal capillaries are very difficult to measure, but are estimated at around 1 and 4mmHg, respectively (Nicolini et al., 1989).

Transfer gradients in pregnancies affected by fetal growth restriction

Maternal and fetal plasma concentration gradients of a variety of substances are altered in FGR. Probably the most rigorous measurements have been of amino acid concentrations (Cetin et al. 1996). Total alpha amino nitrogen levels are higher in maternal plasma and lower in fetal plasma of FGR pregnancies, reflecting such alterations in the concentrations of several specific amino acids. Interestingly, plasma levels of the beta amino acid taurine are also lower in FGR compared with the normally grown fetus (Economides et al. 1989, Cetin et al. 1990). Taurine is particularly important for development of the central nervous system (CNS) (Sturman 1993) and reduced fetal taurine levels are associated with impaired neurological development (Aerts and Van Assche 2002). These altered amino acid differences are also consistent with and probably a reflection of, the lower activity of amino acid transporters in the placenta in FGR (see section on Transporter-mediated transfer in pregnancies affected by FGR).

Despite obvious importance, there have been no measurements of electrical or hydrostatic gradients in FGR. The fact that FGR is often associated with oligohydramnios does suggest there may be some abnormality in the hydrostatic pressure gradient across the placenta (Brownbill and Sibley 2006). Notably, FGR and oligohydramnios are associated with reduced/abnormal spontaneous fetal motility and echogenicity changes in the fetal brain, an early indicator of poor neurological outcome (Rosier-van Dunné et al. 2010).

Diffusional transfer in normal pregnancy

All substances can diffuse across a biological barrier and the placenta is no exception. The rate of net transfer by diffusion of an electroneutral substance (J_{net}) across the placenta, according to Fick's law of diffusion (see Sibley and Boyd 1988), is dependent on the surface area of the barrier available for exchange (A) (effectively the syncytiotrophoblast microvillous membrane—see Fig. 2.1); the thickness of the barrier (l) (syncytiotrophoblast, basement membrane, connective tissue and fetal capillary endothelium—see Fig. 2.1); the diffusion coefficient of the substance in question (D); the concentration gradient between maternal and fetal plasma at the exchange site ($C_m - C_f$). Thus,

$$J_{net} = \frac{AD}{l}(C_m - C_f) \text{ moles/unit time}$$

The importance of the terms on the left side of the equation in determining J_{net} will be dependent on the nature of the substance in question. Small lipophilic substances, such as the respiratory gases, diffuse very rapidly across biological membranes (i.e. have a high value of D) so that the concentration gradient ($C_m - C_f$) and the driving force for diffusion, rapidly becomes dissipated. Transfer by diffusion of these substances is therefore predominantly dependent on maintenance of the concentration gradient for as long as possible across the length of the exchange barrier: this is effectively dependent on blood flow on the two sides and the diffusional transfer of such substances is termed flow limited. This explains why blood flow is so important in determining transfer across the placenta and consequently fetal growth (see section on blood flow below). By contrast, the transfer of larger, hydrophilic substances which diffuse only slowly (low value of D) is much more dependent on the surface area and thickness of the barrier, as the concentration gradient will only be very slowly dissipated. The diffusional transfer of such substances (which include glucose and amino acids) is said to be membrane limited and they may be described as having low permeability across the placenta.

Although diffusion undoubtedly takes place through the plasma membranes that constitute the placental barrier, at rates dependent on substance lipophilicity, there is good evidence for a paracellular (extracellular water filled) route of transfer across the placenta (Fig. 2.2). This is particularly important for the transfer of hydrophilic substances (Atkinson et al. 2006). The morphological correlate of this route is controversial, not least because of the syncytial nature of the syncytiotrophoblast, which does not have the intercellular route of other epithelia. However, there is evidence that areas of syncytial denudation and consequent fibrinoid deposition, as found in all placentas, provide at least one route for paracellular transfer across the human placenta (Brownbill et al. 1995).

Diffusional transfer in pregnancies affected by fetal growth restriction
Diffusional transfer of flow limited substances will be affected by abnormalities in uterine and umbilical blood flow, as defined in FGR and further described below. As regards membrane limited substances, stereological and morphometric studies of the delivered placenta at term show that the surface area for exchange can be reduced and barrier thickness increased in FGR (Mayhew et al. 2004) suggesting that permeability of the FGR placenta is attenuated. In a mouse model of FGR, placental surface area is reduced and trophoblast thickness increased, concomitant with the onset of growth restriction. Compared to wild type litter mates, the permeability of these affected placentas to inert hydrophilic tracers is also reduced (Sibley et al. 2004), suggesting that a change in exchange barrier architecture is an important component of the FGR placental phenotype.

Blood flow in normal pregnancy
The importance of uterine and umbilical blood flow to the placenta for the supply and extraction of nutrients and waste products is emphasised in the discussion of diffusion above. As well as rate of flow, the geometry of the two circulations, relative to each other, will also be important for placental transfer capacity and efficiency. The most efficient arrangement is a countercurrent one, where flow in the circulations on either side of the barrier is in opposition; the least efficient is a concurrent arrangement where the flows are

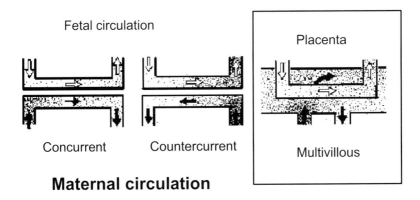

Fig. 2.3. Fetal and maternal blood flow within the human placenta. 'Multivillous pool flow' is multidirectional combining more classic concurrent and countercurrent schemes.

in the same direction either side of the barrier. The human placenta appears to have an arrangement intermediate between these two extremes. Blood jetting into the intervillous space from the spiral arteries on the maternal side results in multidirectional flow at the exchange barrier on this side, while that on the fetal side is linear (Fig. 2.3): this arrangement has been termed 'multivillous pool flow' (Burton et al. 2006).

Blood flow in pregnancies affected by fetal growth restriction
Doppler ultrasound velocimetry has shown abnormal blood flow patterns in both uterine and umbilical circulations in FGR (Karsdorp et al. 1994, Aardema et al. 2001). The higher resistance to flow on the maternal side in FGR is most likely to be explained by retained spiral arteriole contractility as a result of inadequate conversion into low resistance vessels by invading trophoblasts, an early stage of pregnancy (Brosens et al. 2011). However, confirmation is lacking. It is also implied that abnormal umbilical artery Doppler waveforms reflect both abnormal placental villous morphology and abnormal regulation of flow in resistance vessels such as the chorionic plate arteries (Mills et al. 2005, Macara et al. 1996). Although umbilical artery Doppler measurements have proved to be useful in the management of high-risk pregnancies, such as with FGR, neither uterine nor umbilical velocimetry can reliably predict disease or its progression (Karsdorp et al. 1994, Aardema et al. 2001). With oxygen transfer across the placenta being flow limited, uncompensated reductions in blood flow through either utero- or feto-placental circulations can result in placental and fetal hypoxia. Some fetuses affected by FGR show asymmetric growth (Al-Riyami et al. 2011), or head sparing—thought to result from diversion of blood to the head in an attempt to maintain oxygen supply to the brain.

Transporter-mediated transfer in normal pregnancy
There are a panoply of transporter proteins inserted into the maternal facing microvillous plasma membrane (MVM) and fetal facing basal plasma membrane (BPM) of the syncytiotrophoblast (see Figs. 2.1 and 2.2), which catalyse the selective transfer of a wide

variety of solutes—both nutrients and products of metabolism (see Atkinson et al. 2006, Jansson et al. 2009, Desforges and Sibley 2010). The mechanisms by which transfer is accomplished, via transporters, can be illustrated using glucose, amino acids and Ca^{2+} as examples.

In the fetus, glucose is a primary energy source, with its fetal plasma concentration generally lower than that in maternal plasma, providing a gradient for transfer by diffusion. However, the rate of glucose transfer is greater than that expected from diffusion alone prompting a range of investigations to finally confirm its facilitated diffusion through a transporter-protein-mediated pathway (Johnson and Smith 1985, Bissonnette et al. 1981). Such facilitated diffusion also utilises the concentration gradient as the driving force for transfer. Glucose transport in mammalian tissues in general is mediated by the *GLUT* gene family of facilitated diffusion transporters (Joost and Thorens 2001). GLUT1 is expressed in both MVM and BPM and appears to be the major transporter of glucose in the human placenta (Jansson et al. 1993).

Amino acids are required by the fetus for energetic, catabolic and homeostatic purposes. Umbilical cord plasma concentrations of most amino acids are higher than maternal concentrations (Cetin et al. 1996). Furthermore, placental tissue concentrations of amino acids are higher than in both fetal and maternal plasma (Philipps et al. 1978). Net transfer of amino acids to the fetus by diffusion is therefore not possible: energy is required to transport them into the syncytiotrophoblast against the concentration gradient across the MVM. There are generally two systems of amino acid transporters in the MVM—those that co-transport Na^+ with the amino acid (Na^+-dependent systems) and those that do not (Na^+-independent systems) (Christensen 1982). Na^+-dependent amino acid transporters are secondary active transporters that do not directly utilise adenosine triphosphate (ATP). Instead, they harness the active energy of the $Na^+/K^+/ATPase$, creating the Na^+ gradient. It is the energy stored in this Na^+ gradient that is used to transport the amino acids against their concentration gradient (Sibley and Boyd 1988). Good examples of this kind of transporter are system A, which mediates transfer of short chain neutral amino acids such as alanine, glycine and serine and system β/TauT, which transfers taurine. It is not clear what the driving force is for the transport of amino acids across MVM against their concentration gradient by Na^+-independent transporters, though trans-stimulation is the most likely explanation. For example, system L, which mediates leucine transfer, may be trans-stimulated by high intracellular concentrations of another neutral amino acid, such as the system A substrates glycine and serine (Jansson et al. 1998).

Although it is not entirely certain how amino acids exit the syncytiotrophoblast, across the BPM towards the fetus, there is increasing evidence that amino acid exchangers in the BPM may function to take up amino acids required in lower quantities by the fetus in exchange for placental amino acids, for which the fetus has a higher metabolic demand (Cleal et al. 2011). It is also possible that non-mediated diffusion across BPM may contribute to the exit of neutral amino acids from the syncytiotrophoblast towards the fetus, down the concentration gradient from syncytiotrophoblast cytosol to fetal plasma.

The transfer of Ca^{2+} by the placenta is essential for fetal bone mineralisation: fetal accretion of Ca^{2+} increases exponentially over the last third of pregnancy, concomitant with the development of the fetal skeleton (Comar 1956). In all species where it has been measured, including humans, umbilical plasma Ca^{2+} concentrations are higher than those in maternal plasma, suggesting that active, energy-utilising processes are required for net transfer of the cation (Atkinson et al. 2006). Evidence suggests that Ca^{2+} transport across the placenta is likely to involve three main steps (reviewed in Atkinson et al. 2006, Desforges and Sibley 2010): (1) diffusion into the syncytiotrophoblast from maternal plasma down the electrochemical gradient through epithelial Ca^{2+} channels of the transient receptor potential (TRP) gene family; (2) transfer across the syncytiotrophoblast cytoplasm bound to a calcium binding protein (Glazier et al. 1992); or (3) active extrusion into the fetal compartment via plasma membrane Ca^{2+}-ATPase (PMCA) localised to the BPM (Fisher et al. 1987).

Transporter-mediated transfer in pregnancies affected by fetal growth restriction
The expression and activity of a wide range of transporters has been measured in placentas from FGR pregnancies and it is clear that there are major effects of the disease on this mode of exchange compared with normal pregnancy (see Sibley 2009 for detailed review). However, the effects are both transporter and location specific. For example, GLUT expression and activity in MVM and BPM are not altered in FGR (Jansson et al. 1993, 2002); system A and system β/TauT amino acid transporter activity is decreased in the MVM but not BPM (Norberg et al. 1998, Jansson et al. 2002); system L amino acid transporter activity is reduced in both MVM and BPM (Jansson et al. 1998); and PMCA expression and activity in the BPM is actually increased in FGR (Strid et al. 2003). This range of reported effects might reflect the following: (1) the spectrum of disease covered by the term FGR, with different severities of placental dysfunction, and/or (2) a mix of causative and adaptive effects (e.g. decreased placental system A transporter activity leading to reduced amino acid transport and reduced fetal growth in the first instance and reduced Ca^{2+} transfer early in pregnancy leading to placental PMCA over-activity in the latter). There is evidence from both human and animal studies to support the proposition that abnormal placental transporter activity can be both causative and adaptive in relation to FGR (Sibley et al. 2010).

As a marker of placental dysfunction, MVM system A amino acid transporter activity may provide robust indication. In five separate studies of placentas from small for gestational age or FGR pregnancies, its activity in the MVM was found to be reduced (Dicke and Henderson 1988, Glazier et al. 1992, Mahendran et al. 1993, Harrington et al. 1999, Jansson et al. 2002) (though one of the studies only found the reduction in preterm deliveries and not at term, Jansson et al. 2002). Moreover, placentas from non-growing adolescents, who have a greater risk of FGR than their growing counterparts, also have reduced system A activity in placental tissue (Hayward et al. 2011). However, the impact and significance of this finding is yet to be established.

As discussed, placental taurine transfer and fetal taurine levels are reduced in FGR, to the potential detriment of neurological development. Although the links between placental taurine and infant neurodisability require further research, placental taurine levels, measured after delivery, could be used as a biomarker for neurodevelopmental risk and may also allow

17

neonatal care specialists to tailor the infant's feeding to its taurine needs, providing optimal taurine for the neonatal brain.

Defining placental phenotypes

It is clear that factors that determine the capacity of the placenta to exchange nutrients are substantially altered in FGR. There are additional components of the placental phenotype in this disease including alterations in placental size and shape (Salafia et al. 2006, Toal et al. 2007) and alterations in hormone production by the placenta (Bersinger and Odegard 2004). However, what remains uncertain is whether all of these components are always altered in every case of FGR or whether, more likely, there is a spectrum with more components affected when growth restriction is most severe. This is a topic of ongoing research, but knowing the components of the phenotype will only improve our understanding of the aetiology and perhaps diagnosis of FGR and other pregnancy diseases. In addition to the now classic measurements of placental hormones and Doppler velocimetry, new tools and in utero biomarkers are undoubtedly required to achieve this goal, ideally ones which can non-invasively determine the structural and functional phenotypes of the abnormal placenta.

Understanding the aetiology of pregnancy disease

As pregnancy diseases are multifactorial, the aetiology of any particular case is unclear. Although classic pathological examination can be used to identify an underlying placental cause (see Chapter 1), cases with more dysfunctional phenotypes may ultimately be missed. Warrander et al. (2012) studied the structure and function of placentas delivered within 7 days of women reporting reduced fetal movements (RFM). Although RFM is linked to both FGR and stillbirth, no previous study had determined its association with placental phenotypes of disease. It was found that women who reported RFM had smaller placentas than those with normal outcomes. Moreover, histopathologically these placentas had more areas of infarction, increased proliferation but no change in apoptotic index. System A amino acid transporter activity was also reduced, suggesting that function as well as structure is inherently different in these pregnancies. Interestingly, for all phenotypes, their degree of intensity was exaggerated in women with RFM of worse pregnancy outcome (i.e. stillbirth, preterm birth, small for gestational age or term admission to the neonatal intensive care unit).

These data suggest that biomarkers of placental function, following presentation of RFM, may have utility in diagnosing women at highest risk of fetal compromise, allowing a window of opportunity for clinical intervention. This was further investigated by Dutton et al. (2012) who tested the hypothesis that markers of placental insufficiency might improve detection of poor outcome following RFM. They found that maternal serum concentrations (in samples taken soon after reported RFM) of three placentally derived hormones, human chorionic gonadotrophin, human placental lactogen and progesterone, were reduced in women of poor pregnancy outcome. In multivariate analysis, circulating human placental lactogen was also independently associated. These data support the concept that a basket of measures of placental disease phenotype may hold value in obstetric diagnosis.

Improving the diagnosis of pregnancy disease

The concept that tests of placental structure and function in utero might improve early diagnosis of pregnancy complications has been put into practice in at least two centres worldwide (Toronto and Manchester), in the form of placental clinics (Toal et al. 2007, Acharya et al. 2012). Within these antenatal units, ultrasound assessment of placental morphology, Doppler ultrasound on the uterine artery and maternal serum screening are being used with increasing success in predicting adverse pregnancy outcomes. Nevertheless, it is clear that these approaches need to be complemented with more sophisticated techniques to fully appreciate all aspects of aberrant placental phenotype. In this regard, magnetic resonance imaging (MRI) may be of clinical value. MRI can potentially be used to detect a number of different aspects of placental structure and function, simultaneously and non-invasively. This concept is supported by reports of correlations between MRI variables measured in utero and placental structure measured following delivery (Wright et al. 2011). Moreover, differences in MRI measurements in normal versus FGR pregnancies, in placental shape, size and blood flow (Damodaram et al. 2010), propose that functional MRI might also be possible (Hibbeln et al. 2012). This is further supported by demonstration of the feasibility of using MRI to investigate placental oxygenation (Huen et al. 2013), which could be a useful tool for detecting placental and fetal hypoxia.

Conclusion

In this chapter, we have sought to outline the placental phenotypes recently shown to be associated with pregnancy diseases, using FGR as an example. Elsewhere in this book, current knowledge of how different aspects of placental structure, morphology and function are, or might be, correlated with neurodisability is discussed. Our contention is that all of this information needs to be put together to derive a placental phenotype (or phenotypes) associated with childhood neurodisability. This could then be used to both improve postnatal identification of those pregnancies associated with placental dysfunction and provide diagnostic biomarkers of those at risk. To be able to use placental phenotypes in diagnosis needs further improvements in in utero detection. MRI is one technique showing promise in this regard, as further detailed in Chapter 8, especially as combined placental and fetal brain imaging seems feasible, for direct connections between placental phenotype and brain disease (Girard et al. 2010).

REFERENCES

Aardema MW, Oosterhof H, Timmer A, Van Rooy I, Aarnoudse JG (2001) Uterine artery Doppler flow and uteroplacental vascular pathology in normal pregnancies and pregnancies complicated by pre-eclampsia and small for gestational age fetuses. *Placenta* 22: 405–411. doi: http://dx.doi.org/10.1053/plac.2001.0676

Acharya G, Albrecht C, Benton SJ et al. (2012) IFPA Meeting 2011 workshop report I: Placenta: Predicting future health; roles of lipids in the growth and development of feto-placental unit; placental nutrient sensing; placental research to solve clinical problems - A translational approach. *Placenta* 33: S4–S8. doi: http://dx.doi.org/10.1016/j.placenta.2011.11.015

Aerts L, Van Assche FA (2002) Taurine and taurine-deficiency in the perinatal period. *J Perinat Med* 30: 281–286. doi: http://dx.doi.org/10.1515/jpm.2002.040

Al-Riyami N, Walker MG, Proctor LK, Yinon Y, Windrim RC, Kingdom JC (2011) Utility of head/abdomen circumference ratio in the evaluation of severe early-onset intrauterine growth restriction. *J Obstet Gynaecol Can* 33: 715–719.

Atkinson DE, Boyd RDH, Sibley CP (2006) Placental transfer (Chapter 52). In: Neill JD, editor. *Knobil and Neill's Physiology of Reproduction*, 3rd ed. Amsterdam: Elsevier.

Baschat AA (2011) Neurodevelopment following fetal growth restriction and its relationship with antepartum parameters of placental dysfunction. *Ultrasound Obstet Gynecol* 37: 501–514. doi: http://dx.doi.org/10.1002/uog.9008

Bersinger NA, Odegard RA (2004) Second- and third-trimester serum levels of placental proteins in pre-eclampsia and small-for-gestational age pregnancies. *Acta Obstet Gynecol Scand* 83: 37–45. doi: http://dx.doi.org/10.1111/j.1600-0412.2004.00277.x

Bissonnette JM, Black JA, Wickham WK, Acott KM (1981) Glucose uptake into plasma membrane vesicles from the maternal surface of human placenta. *J Membr Biol* 58: 75–80. doi: http://dx.doi.org/10.1007/bf01871036

Brosens I, Pijnenborg R, Vercruysse L, Romero R (2011) The "Great Obstetrical Syndromes" are associated with disorders of deep placentation. *Am J Obstet Gynecol* 204: 193–201. Doi: http://dx.doi.org/10.1016/j.ajog.2010.08.009

Brownbill P, Edwards D, Jones C et al. (1995) Mechanisms of alphafetoprotein transfer in the perfused human placental cotyledon from uncomplicated pregnancy. *J Clin Invest* 96: 2220–2226. Doi: http://dx.doi.org/10.1172/jci118277

Brownbill P, Sibley CP (2006) Regulation of transplacental water transfer: The role of fetoplacental venous tone. *Placenta* 27: 560–567. Doi: http://dx.doi.org/10.1016/j.placenta.2005.08.002

Burton GJ, Kaufmann P, Huppertz B (2006) Anatomy and genesis of the placenta (Chapter 5). In: Neil JD, editor. *Physiology of Reproduction*, 3rd ed. Amsterdam: Elsevier.

Cetin I, Corbetta C, Sereni LP et al. (1990) Umbilical amino acid concentrations in normal and growth-retarded fetuses sampled in utero by cordocentesis. *Am J Obstet Gynecol* 162: 253–261. doi: http://dx.doi.org/10.1016/0002-9378(90)90860-a

Cetin I, Ronzoni S, Marconi AM et al. (1996) Maternal concentrations and fetal-maternal concentration differences of plasma amino acids in normal and intrauterine growth-restricted pregnancies. *Am J Obstet Gynecol* 174: 1575–1583. Doi: http://dx.doi.org/10.1016/s0002-9378(96)70609-9

Christensen HN (1982) Interorgan amino acid nutrition. *Physiol Rev* 62: 1193–1233.

Cleal JK, Glazier JD, Ntani G et al. (2011) Facilitated transporters mediate net efflux of amino acids to the fetus across the basal membrane of the placental syncytiotrophoblast. *J Physiol* 589: 987–997. Doi: http://dx.doi.org/10.1113/jphysiol.2010.198549

Comar CL (1956) Radiocalcium studies in pregnancy. *Ann N Y Acad Sci* 64: 281–298. Doi: http://dx.doi.org/10.1111/j.1749-6632.1956.tb52449.x

Damodaram M, Story L, Eixarch E et al. (2010) Placental MRI in intrauterine fetal growth restriction. *Placenta* 31: 491–498. Doi: http://dx.doi.org/10.1016/j.placenta.2010.03.001

Desforges M, Sibley CP (2009) Placental nutrient supply and fetal growth. *Int J Dev Biol* 54: 377–390.

Dicke JM, Henderson GI (1988) Placental amino acid uptake in normal and complicated pregnancies. *Am J Med Sci* 295: 223–227. Doi: http://dx.doi.org/10.1097/00000441-198803000-00012

Dutton PJ, Warrander LK, Roberts SA et al. (2012) Predictors of poor perinatal outcome following maternal perception of reduced fetal movements – A prospective cohort study. *PLoS One* 7: e39784. Doi: http://dx.doi.org/10.1371/journal.pone.0039784

Economides DL, Nicolaides KH, Gahl WA, Bernardini I, Evans MI (1989) Plasma amino acids in appropriate- and small-for-gestational-age fetuses. *Am J Obstet Gynecol* 161: 1219–1227. Doi: http://dx.doi.org/10.1016/0002-9378(89)90670-4

Fisher GJ, Kelley LK, Smith CH (1987) ATP-dependent calcium transport across basal plasma membranes of human placental trophoblast. *Am J Physiol* 252: C38–C46.

Flexner LB, Gelhorn A (1942) The comparative physiology of placental transfer. *Am J Obstet Gynecol* 43: 965–974.

Girard S, Tremblay L, Lepage M, Sebire G (2010) IL-1 receptor antagonist protects against placental and neurodevelopmental defects induced by maternal inflammation. *J Immunol* 184: 3997–4005. Doi: http://dx.doi.org/10.4049/jimmunol.0903349

Glazier JD, Atkinson DE, Thornburg KL et al. (1992) Gestational changes in Ca2+ transport across rat placenta and mRNA for calbindin9K and Ca(2+)-ATPase. *Am J Physiol* 263: R930–R935.

Greenwood SL, Boyd RD, Sibley CP (1993) Transtrophoblast and microvillus membrane potential difference in mature intermediate human placental villi. *Am J Physiol* 265: C460–C466.

Harrington B, Glazier J, D'Souza S, Sibley C (1999) System A amino acid transporter activity in human placental microvillous membrane vesicles in relation to various anthropometric measurements in appropriate and small for gestational age babies. *Pediatr Res* 45: 810–814. Doi: http://dx.doi.org/10.1203/00006450-199906000-00005

Hayward CE, Greenwood SL, Sibley CP, Baker PN, Challis JR, Jones RL (2011) Effect of maternal age and growth on placental nutrient transport: Potential mechanisms for teenagers' predisposition to small-for-gestational-age birth? *Am J Physiol Endocrinol Metab* 302: E233–E242. Doi: http://dx.doi.org/10.1152/ajpendo.00192.2011

Hibbeln JF, Shors SM, Byrd SE (2012) MRI: Is there a role in obstetrics? *Clin Obstet Gynecol* 55: 352–366.

Huen I, Morris DM, Wright C et al. (2013) *R*1 and *R*2* changes in the human placenta in response to maternal oxygen challenge. *Magn Reson Med* 70(5): 1427–1433. Doi: http://dx.doi.org/10.1002/mrm.24581

Jansson T, Myatt L, Powell TL (2009) The role of trophoblast nutrient and ion transporters in the development of pregnancy complications and adult disease. *Curr Vasc Pharmacol* 7: 521–533. Doi: http://dx.doi.org/10.2174/157016109789043982

Jansson T, Scholtbach V, Powell TL (1998) Placental transport of leucine and lysine is reduced in intrauterine growth restriction. *Pediatr Res* 44: 532–537. Doi: http://dx.doi.org/10.1203/00006450-199810000-00011

Jansson T, Wennergren M, Illsley NP (1993) Glucose transporter protein expression in human placenta throughout gestation and in intrauterine growth retardation. *J Clin Endocrinol Metab* 77: 1554–1562. Doi: http://dx.doi.org/10.1210/jcem.77.6.8263141

Jansson T, Ylven K, Wennergren M, Powell TL (2002) Glucose transport and system A activity in syncytiotrophoblast microvillous and basal plasma membranes in intrauterine growth restriction. *Placenta* 23: 392–399. Doi: http://dx.doi.org/10.1053/plac.2002.0826

Johnson LW, Smith CH (1985) Glucose transport across the basal plasma membrane of human placental syncytiotrophoblast. *Biochim Biophys Acta* 815: 44–50. Doi: http://dx.doi.org/10.1016/0005-2736(85)90472-9

Joost HG, Thorens B (2001) The extended GLUT-family of sugar/polyol transport facilitators: Nomenclature, sequence characteristics, and potential function of its novel members (review). *Mol Membr Biol* 18: 247–256. Doi: http://dx.doi.org/10.1080/09687680110090456

Karsdorp VH, Van Vugt JM, Van Geijn HP et al. (1994) Clinical significance of absent or reversed end diastolic velocity waveforms in umbilical artery. *Lancet* 344: 1664–1668. Doi: http://dx.doi.org/10.1016/s0140-6736(94)90457-x

Macara L, Kingdom JC, Kaufmann P et al. (1996) Structural analysis of placental terminal villi from growth-restricted pregnancies with abnormal umbilical artery Doppler waveforms. *Placenta* 17: 37–48. Doi: http://dx.doi.org/10.1016/s0143-4004(05)80642-3

Mahendran D, Donnai P, Glazier JD, D'Souza SW, Boyd RD, Sibley CP (1993) Amino acid (system A) transporter activity in microvillous membrane vesicles from the placentas of appropriate and small for gestational age babies. *Pediatr Res* 34: 661–665. Doi: http://dx.doi.org/10.1203/00006450-199311000-00019

Mayhew TM, Wijesekara J, Baker PN, Ong SS (2004) Morphometric evidence that villous development and fetoplacental angiogenesis are compromised by intrauterine growth restriction but not by pre-eclampsia. *Placenta* 25: 829–833. Doi: http://dx.doi.org/10.1016/j.placenta.2004.04.011

Mills TA, Wareing M, Bugg GJ, Greenwood SL, Baker PN (2005) Chorionic plate artery function and Doppler indices in normal pregnancy and intrauterine growth restriction. *Eur J Clin Invest* 35: 758–764. Doi: http://dx.doi.org/10.1111/j.1365-2362.2005.01577.x

Nicolini U, Fisk NM, Talbert DG et al. (1989) Intrauterine manometry: Technique and application to fetal pathology. *Prenat Diagn* 9: 243–254. Doi: http://dx.doi.org/10.1002/pd.1970090404

Norberg S, Powell TL, Jansson T (1998) Intrauterine growth restriction is associated with a reduced activity of placental taurine transporters. *Pediatr Res* 44: 233–238. Doi: http://dx.doi.org/10.1203/00006450-199808000-00016

Philipps AF, Holzman IR, Teng C, Battaglia FC (1978) Tissue concentrations of free amino acids in term human placentas. *Am J Obstet Gynecol* 131: 881–887.

Reik W, Constancia M, Fowden A et al. (2003) Regulation of supply and demand for maternal nutrients in mammals by imprinted genes. *J Physiol* 547: 35–44. http://dx.doi.org/10.1111/j.1469-7793.2003.00035.x

Rosier-Van Dunné FM, Van Wezel-Meijler G, Bakker MP, Odendaal HJ, De Vries JI (2010) Fetal general movements and brain sonography in a population at risk for preterm birth. *Early Hum Dev* 86: 107–111. Doi: http://dx.doi.org/10.1016/j.earlhumdev.2010.01.026

Salafia CM, Charles AK, Maas EM (2006) Placenta and fetal growth restriction. *Clin Obstet Gynecol* 49: 236–256. Doi: http://dx.doi.org/10.1097/00003081-200606000-00007

Sibley CP (2009) Understanding placental nutrient transfer – why bother? New biomarkers of fetal growth. *J Physiol* 587: 3431–3440. Doi: http://dx.doi.org/10.1113/jphysiol.2009.172403

Sibley CP, Boyd RDH (1988) Control of transfer across the mature placenta. In: Clarke JR, editor. *Oxford Reviews of Reproductive Biology*. Oxford: Oxford University Press.

Sibley CP, Brownbill P, Dilworth M, Glazier JD (2010) Review: Adaptation in placental nutrient supply to meet fetal growth demand: implications for programming. *Placenta* Suppl 31: S70–S74.

Sibley CP, Coan PM, Ferguson-Smith AC et al. (2004) Placental-specific insulin-like growth factor 2 (Igf2) regulates the diffusional exchange characteristics of the mouse placenta. *Proc Natl Acad Sci U S A* 101: 8204–8208. Doi: http://dx.doi.org/10.1073/pnas.0402508101

Strid H, Bucht E, Jansson T, Wennergren M, Powell TL (2003) ATP dependent Ca^{2+} transport across basal membrane of human syncytiotrophoblast in pregnancies complicated by intrauterine growth restriction or diabetes. *Placenta* 24: 445–452.Doi: http://dx.doi.org/10.1053/plac.2002.0941

Sturman JA (1993) Taurine in development. *Physiol Rev* 73: 119–147.

Toal M, Chan C, Fallah S et al. (2007) Usefulness of a placental profile in high-risk pregnancies. *Am J Obstet Gynecol* 196: 363.e1–363.e7. Doi: http://dx.doi.org/10.1016/j.ajog.2006.10.897

Warrander LK, Batra G, Bernatavicius G et al. (2012) Maternal perception of reduced fetal movements is associated with altered placental structure and function. *PLoS One* 7: e34851. Doi: http://dx.doi.org/10.1371/journal.pone.0034851

Wright C, Morris DM, Baker PN et al. (2011) Magnetic resonance imaging relaxation time measurements of the placenta at 1.5 T. *Placenta* 32: 1010–1015. Doi: http://dx.doi.org/10.1016/j.placenta.2011.07.008

3
ABERRANT PLACENTAL ENDOCRINOLOGY, FETAL GROWTH AND NEURODEVELOPMENT

Jayne Charnock and Melissa Westwood

The placenta is a major source of steroid and protein hormones, some of which are unique to pregnancy (see Fig. 3.1). It is also responsible for modulating fetal exposure to hormones produced by the mother. Aberrations in these functions may directly influence fetal neuro-development, as both placental and maternal hormones impact upon the fetal brain. Likewise, abnormal placental hormone production and/or metabolism may also influence fetal growth.

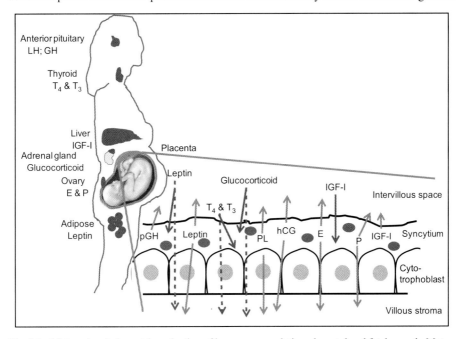

Fig. 3.1. Maternal and placental production of hormones regulating placental and fetal growth. Maternal hormones and their sites of production are shown in red. Solid red arrows indicate action in placenta, whereas dotted red arrows denote hormones that are transferred across the placenta into the fetal circulation. Hormones produced by the placenta are shown in blue; all have functions within the placenta and their secretion into the maternal and fetal circulations is depicted by blue arrows. A colour version of this figure can be seen in the plate section at the end of the book.

Overall, there is a strong correlation between placental weight and fetal growth, with most low birthweight infants having a smaller placenta (Godfrey et al. 1996). Birthweight is a well-recognized marker of the risk of developing disease and disorders, for example, obesity, diabetes and hypertension in later life (Gluckman et al. 2008). Likewise, mental health is programmed in utero, again with lower birthweight associated with later affective and cognitive disorders (reviewed in Shenkin et al. 2004, Hayes and Sharif 2009, Schlotz and Phillips 2009).

This chapter considers the role of key hormones produced (estrogen, progesterone, human chorionic gonadotrophin [hCG], human placental lactogen [hPL], placental GH [pGH], leptin and insulin-like growth factor [IGF]) and/or handled by the human placenta (leptin, IGF, glucocorticoids and thyroid hormones), paying particular attention to placental function, fetal growth and fetal neurological development.

Estrogen and progesterone
In early pregnancy, the corpus luteum is responsible for the production of the steroids, estrogen and progesterone. From week 6 of gestation, the placenta takes over this role, increasing their synthesis exponentially thereafter. Within the human placenta, syncytiotrophoblast expresses the enzyme aromatase, which converts androgens, derived from both the mother and the fetus, into estrogen. All three estrogens, estradiol, estrone and estriol, are produced, though mainly the latter due to predominance of its precursor 16α-DHEA sulfate, derived from the fetal liver and adrenals (Ackerman and Carr 2002). Estrogens are thought to be involved in the maternal cardiovascular adaptations to pregnancy and they are also potent dilators of uterine vessels, enhancing utero-placental blood flow and ultimately, transfer of nutrients to the fetus. Less is known about whether they have a direct role within placenta, though they can stimulate leptin expression (Henson and Castracane 2006) and are thought to regulate trophoblast differentiation (Rama et al. 2004), extravillous trophoblast invasion and vascular remodeling (Albrecht et al. 2006).

Progesterone production, again by the syncytiotrophoblast, is dependent on maternal and fetal cholesterol, as unlike other steroid producing glands it is unable to synthesize this precursor de novo. The progesterone secreted into the maternal blood stream has a number of actions within the uterus, including stimulating further differentiation of the endometrium and suppressing myometrial contractions, which are essential for the maintenance of pregnancy. It is also involved in the immune and metabolic adaptation to pregnancy. Progesterone attenuates the action of insulin in peripheral tissues and mediates an increase in maternal appetite both directly by stimulating expression of hypothalamic peptides and indirectly by attenuating the effect of leptin at the hypothalamus (Newbern and Freemark 2011).

Placentally derived estrogen and progesterone contribute to the level of these steroids in the fetal circulation and fetal exposure increases as pregnancy progresses. Estrogen and progesterone receptors, both of which belong to the intracellular steroid hormone receptor superfamily, function as transcription factors regulating responsive genes. These receptors are expressed in the developing brain (Gonzalez et al. 2007, Wagner 2008) and are therefore likely to influence fetal brain development. Indeed, both hormones have neurotropic and neuroprotective actions and are involved in neuronal differentiation, synapse formation and cognitive function (Beyer 1999, Wagner 2008). At birth, the neonate is subjected to an abrupt withdrawal of these placental hormones, which has no consequence for the infant born at term, but may be detrimental for the continued neurodevelopment of the preterm infant. In keeping with this hypothesis, data from a recent study suggest that postnatal estrogen and progesterone replacement may improve neurodevelopmental outcomes of extremely preterm, low-birthweight infants (Trotter et al. 2012).

Human chorionic gonadotrophin

Human chorionic gonadotrophin (hCG) is produced by the syncytiotrophoblast of the human placenta within the first 7 days of fertilization; cytotrophoblast, specifically extravillous cytotrophoblast, also produces glycosylated variants, so-called hyperglycosylated hCG (hCG-H). hCG and hCG-H have a similar structure to luteinizing hormone (LH) and thus bind to the same receptor, the LH/hCG receptor (LH/hCG-R). Classically, hCG is known for "rescuing" the corpus luteum and maintaining ovarian production of progesterone, despite falling levels of LH. This role continues until 7 weeks' gestation, when the placenta facilitates steroid synthesis. Although the subsequent production of hCG and hCG-H declines, they remain present at high concentrations suggesting further roles in pregnancy.

hCG promotes the growth and development of the placenta as it stimulates cytotrophoblast differentiation into syncytiotrophoblast (Pidoux et al. 2012). It also supports spiral arteriole angiogenesis to ensure an optimal utero-placental blood supply (Zygmunt et al. 2002). hCG-H stimulates cytotrophoblast proliferation and migration and levels notably correlate with decidual and uterine microvessel invasion (Chen et al. 2012). Consequently, placental volume and vascularity is associated with maternal hCG levels in the first trimester and low levels are linked to fetal growth restriction (FGR) (Krantz et al. 2004). Similarly, low levels of hCG-H are associated with an increased risk of developing pre-eclampsia (Bahado-Singh et al. 2002).

hCG is also present in the fetal circulation, as a result of placental transfer. LH/hCG-R is present in the developing mammalian brain (al-Hader et al. 1997) and in vitro hCG stimulates neuronal differentiation, suggesting a role for hCG in CNS development. Impaired production may therefore provide a direct link between reduced placental size, fetal growth and neurodisability.

Insulin-like growth factors

The IGF system plays a key role in the regulation of fetal and placental growth throughout gestation. Aberrant IGF signaling during pregnancy is associated with poor fetal outcome, both directly, in relation to altered fetal IGF levels and indirectly, as a result of detrimental changes to the essential functions IGFs play in supporting normal placental development and function. The IGF system consists of two signaling peptides, IGF-I and IGF-II, the actions of which are mediated by binding to the type-1 IGF receptor (IGF1R), to promote various cellular functions including proliferation, differentiation and survival. IGF-II is also able to bind to the type-2 IGF receptor (IGF2R), also known as the mannose-6-phosphate receptor, which is thought to be capable of promoting cell turnover and migration, but is primarily understood to act as a clearance receptor for IGF-II (Harris and Westwood 2012). In addition, IGF-II may also bind to the insulin receptor, further modulating cell function (Louvi et al. 1997). The availability of the IGF peptides to bind to these receptors and their biological half-lives is regulated by a family of IGF-binding proteins (IGFBPs) 1–6. They can therefore sequester IGF activity, but during pregnancy their affinity for binding IGFs is reduced, thereby increasing IGF levels available for signaling (Forbes and Westwood 2008). The regulation of fetal IGF expression is also mediated by environmental factors, including maternal nutrition, smoking status and endocrine agents such as insulin, glucocorticoids, hPL and thyroid hormone levels.

During pregnancy, maternal, placental and fetal IGFs all play parts in driving development in utero. While there is currently no evidence that maternal IGFs can themselves cross the placenta to exert direct effects on fetal growth, they are, along with locally produced IGFs, known to mediate almost all aspects of placental growth and functional capacity. Both IGF-I and -II are present in most cell types of the placenta from as early as 6 weeks' gestation and IGF1R is expressed by placental cells ubiquitously, including the trophoblast, villous endothelium and mesenchymal stroma (Han et al. 1996). IGFR2 is also localized to the trophoblast, but may be cleaved to release a soluble form which when bound to IGF-II results in degradation, potentially providing a mechanism for preventing excess IGF-II effects (Harris et al. 2011).

Specifically, *in vitro* studies have demonstrated the importance of IGFs in proliferation and survival of placental cytotrophoblasts and fibroblasts, migration of extravillous trophoblasts, regulation of cytotrophoblast differentiation and modulation of nutrient transport, including the stimulation of glucose and amino acid uptake (Forbes et al. 2008). These effects may be borne out in both human and animal pregnancies in which maternal IGF-I levels, which increase throughout gestation, have been shown to positively correlate with both fetal and placental weight (Luo et al. 2012). In addition, *in vivo* studies have confirmed that enhancing maternal IGF-I and IGF-II leads to improved fetal weight, with enhanced placental glucose transport, nutrient partitioning (IGF-I) and modifications to structure that increase functional capacity (IGF-II) (Sferruzzi-Perri et al. 2008). These findings suggest complementary roles for IGF-I and IGF-II in driving placental exchange to promote fetal growth.

Disordered growth has been related to abnormal expression levels of the IGFBPs. Increased levels of maternal circulating and decidual IGFBP-1 have been described in patients with FGR and pre-eclampsia, the latter suggested as a result of IGFBP-1 inhibition of trophoblast invasion, resulting in poor implantation and spiral artery remodeling (Chard 1994, Agodi et al. 1995, Klauwer et al. 1997).

Levels of fetally derived IGFs are also closely associated with birth outcome. Both IGFs are detected in the fetal circulation from early in gestation, but concentrations of IGF-II are 3–10-fold higher than those of IGF-I, which has led to the suggestion that IGF-II is primarily responsible for fetal growth, although there is a shift toward IGF-I after birth. Levels of newborn cord blood are correlated to birthweight and thus levels are decreased in patients with fetal growth restriction (FGR). Studies of circulating IGFs in dizygotic twins with different birthweights have found that significantly different IGF-I levels are present (the smaller twin expressing the lower level) and the concordant levels observed in monozygotic twins suggest an element of genetic determination (Westwood et al. 2001).

Much of our understanding of the importance of IGFs in fetal development comes from gene expression studies in mice. Deletion of either the *Igf1* or *Igf2* genes retards fetal growth to about 60% of wild-type animals (most *Igf1* mutants die shortly after birth, although *Igf2* null pups grow normally postnatally) (DeChiara et al. 1990, Baker et al. 1993). An additive effect is seen in double mutants which have birthweights 30% that of normal pups. The only reported human case of a mutation in *Igf1* also resulted in a FGR phenotype (Woods et al. 1996). While *Igf1* deletion has no effect on placental weight, *Igf2* knockout mice have placentas that are 25% smaller, which again highlights the importance of this factor in driving placental growth. The placental specific *Igf2* or *P0* knockout mouse has further demonstrated the essential role placental IGF-II plays in development, since in this mutant reduced placental growth is followed by reduced fetal growth (thought to be a result of a thickened placental exchange barrier and therefore reduced nutrient diffusion) (Constancia et al. 2002). Manipulation of receptor genes also results in an altered fetal outcome. *Igf1r* deletion produces a more severe growth restricted phenotype than either *Igf1* or *Igf2* mutants, but conversely deletion of *Igr2r* results in fetal and placental overgrowth, which is likely to be a result of fetal IGF-II over-expression due to impaired clearance by the receptor. Further genetic studies into the roles of IGFBPs confirm clinical observations in human pregnancies, that elevated levels of IGFBP-1 or IGFBP-3 in pregnant mice result in a growth restricted phenotype.

Typically IGF-induced changes in birthweight are accompanied by abnormalities of development of individual mouse fetal tissues, including delayed ossification, thinned skin, hypoplasia of respiratory muscles, cardiac abnormalities as well as decreased brain size and postnatal brain growth (Laviola et al. 2008). In general, IGF-I is an essential component of brain development and promotes nerve cell metabolism, neurogenesis, myelination, vascularization and acts as a neuronal survival factor, among other functions. Crucially, a number of neurodegenerative diseases such as Alzheimer and motor neuron disease are accompanied by reduced circulating IGF-I levels (Russo et al. 2005). Although research into the relevance of altered IGF during pregnancy on fetal brain development is limited, one study reported reductions in cerebellar and hypothalamic weights following maternal nutrient restriction, known to cause aberrations in IGF levels (Chowen et al. 2002). Given the importance of IGFs in fetal and placental growth, the implications of poor pregnancy outcome on neurological outcome and the role that the IGF axis plays directly in driving brain development, it is likely that this system is essential for appropriate in utero programming of the neonatal CNS.

Placental growth hormone and placental lactogen
In humans, the growth hormone gene locus has evolved and diverged from a common ancestor and is now part of a cluster of five genes that encode growth hormone expressed by the anterior pituitary gland (*GH-N*), placental GH (*GH-V*) and placental lactogen (*hCS-L, -A* and *-B*). Despite strong gene and protein homology across the cluster, regulation of gene expression is tissue specific and the proteins have different functions. Transcription of *GH-V* is specific to placenta, in particular the syncytiotrophoblast and gives rise to two isoforms of pGH that are very similar in sequence and structure to pituitary GH (pGH).

pGH produced by the placenta stimulates maternal lipolysis and gluconeogenesis in the liver and is the main effector of the relative maternal insulin insensitivity that occurs during pregnancy as a mechanism for mobilizing maternal nutrients to maximize their availability for transfer to the fetus. Human placental lactogen (hPL) also contributes to this process. hPL is produced by syncytiotrophoblast (the mature hormone derived from each of the three genes is identical) and levels within the maternal circulation increase rapidly from early in the first trimester. hPL probably plays a role in the induction of maternal hyperphagia and weight gain (Freemark 2006) and is also important in the maternal pancreatic adaptation to pregnancy-induced insulin resistance (Brelje et al. 1993). In addition, pGH and possibly hPL take over from pGH in the regulation of maternal IGF-I, as described above.

In early pregnancy, maternal levels of pGH, but not hPL, are associated with fetal growth rate. However, at term placental expression of pGH and hPL is reduced in pregnancies complicated by FGR (Caufriez et al. 1993, Mannik et al. 2010, Koutsaki et al. 2011); currently, it is not clear whether this is a direct cause or effect of the associated reduction in placental growth. The human placenta expresses the receptor for growth hormone (GHR), which suggests that pGH may also have a role in regulating placental growth and/or function. *GHR* contains a common polymorphism, which leads to the deletion of exon 3 (Stallings-Mann et al. 1996) and altered sensitivity to pituitary-derived GH (Dos et al. 2004) and presumably, pGH. Interestingly, placental weight and fetal weight are affected by GHR genotype, with infants homozygous for deletion having smaller placentas and birthweights.

pGH is not found within the fetal circulation, whereas hPL is present from early gestation and there is widespread expression of the receptor hPLR within fetal tissues. As a result of the numerous *in vitro* studies showing that hPL has both mitogenic and anabolic actions, it is proposed as a regulator of fetal growth and development, potentially through the stimulation of fetal IGF production.

Leptin

Leptin is a peptide hormone produced by white adipose tissue in response to feeding; therefore, levels in the circulation reflect fat mass. Leptin has pleiotropic effects but is well recognized as a signal of satiety by acting on neurons in the hypothalamus, via the leptin receptor, reducing food intake and increasing energy expenditure.

Leptin is produced in abundance by the human placenta. Its level in the maternal circulation begins to rise in the first trimester and remains elevated, relative to non-pregnant women, thereafter. A soluble form of the receptor, generated by proteolytic cleavage of its extracellular domain, increases with advancing gestation. This increase, along with the development of central leptin resistance, is thought to represent a mechanism for enhancing leptin levels without activating hypothalamic pathways to suppress appetite. Interestingly, maternal leptin levels in the first trimester are not associated with infant birthweight at term (Hedley et al. 2009), whereas high levels of maternal leptin in late pregnancy are correlated with impaired fetal growth (Mise et al. 2007).

The leptin receptor is also present in human placenta. Both villous and extravillous trophoblast expresses the receptor, which suggests that leptin has a role in regulating placental growth and function. Indeed, *in vitro* studies have shown that leptin stimulates villous trophoblast proliferation and survival (Maymo et al. 2011), hCG production and activity of the amino acid transporter system A (von Versen-Hoynck et al. 2009). In explants derived from placentas of obese women, syncytiotrophoblast expression of the leptin receptor and leptin-stimulated system A activity are reduced, suggesting that maternal hyperleptinemia may result in placental leptin resistance and impaired placental function (Farley et al. 2010).

In addition to these placental effects, there is considerable evidence to suggest that maternal and placental leptin may contribute to the level of leptin in the fetus and therefore have a direct impact on fetal development. Studies in rats have shown that maternal leptin can be transferred across the placenta and into the fetal circulation, through a mechanism involving the soluble form of the leptin receptor. Data obtained using the villous trophoblast cell line, [BeWo], suggest that this pathway may also operate in humans. The concentration of leptin in the umbilical vein is significantly higher than that in the umbilical artery and, following birth, there is a rapid decline in the circulating level in the newborn infant. Moreover, cord levels reflect maternal body mass index as fetuses of lean mothers have lower cord leptin levels than those of obese women (Catalano et al. 2009) and in studies of FGR in both singleton and twin pregnancies, decreased placental leptin expression is associated with a decrease in leptin in the umbilical vein (Lea et al. 2000, Sooranna et al. 2001a, 2001b).

Within the fetus, leptin probably regulates many aspects of development, including development of the brain. Leptin can cross the blood–brain barrier from early on in fetal development and the leptin receptor is expressed throughout the developing brain. In rodents, leptin stimulates neurogenesis and axon growth in the fetal cerebral cortex and therefore has the potential to influence the establishment of circuits involved in motor and cognitive processes. Animal studies have shown that offspring of undernourished mothers have impaired neurodevelopment (Bouret 2010), whereas maternal obesity leads to leptin resistance in the offspring and consequently reduced hypothalamic response to leptin, in terms of food intake, during critical periods of development (Kirk et al. 2009). It is tempting to speculate that other aspects of brain development will be similarly affected. Indeed, other animal models of leptin resistance and leptin deficiency, have impaired hippocampal synaptic plasticity and they perform poorly in tasks designed to test spatial memory (Harvey et al. 2006).

In humans, the concentration of leptin in cord blood is correlated to head circumference, which supports the hypothesis that leptin also influences human brain development (Bouret 2010). Moreover, young children with low leptin levels, for example, as a result of mutations in the leptin gene, have delayed neurocognitive development. Administration of physiological doses of recombinant leptin improves their rate of cognitive development (Paz-Filho et al. 2008, 2011), which suggests leptin as a potential therapy for overcoming adverse developmental programming, induced by suboptimal maternal and/or placental leptin production.

Glucocorticoids

Glucocorticoids (i.e. cortisol) are synthesized in the zona fasiculata of the adrenal cortex under the influence of corticotrophin-releasing hormone and adrenocorticotropic hormone produced by the hypothalamus and anterior pituitary gland respectively. In adult life, their principle role is to enhance glucose production through the regulation of protein, carbohydrate and lipid production, though they are also involved in modulating the immune and stress responses. The fetus requires glucocorticoids for normal development of the brain (and other organs); however, excess exposure is detrimental to neuron function and brain structure (French et al. 1999), as well as fetal growth (Weinstock 2005) and can have long-term consequences for the offspring, including altered neurophysiology, affecting both cognition and behavior and increased susceptibility to adult-onset disease (Harris and Seckl 2011, Kapoor et al. 2008).

The fetus is protected from maternal glucocorticoids by the placenta, which expresses the enzyme 11β-hydroxysteroid dehydrogenase 2 (11β-HSD2) in increasing abundance as gestation progresses. This enzyme metabolizes the majority of maternal glucocorticoids into inactive cortisone and therefore only 10%–20% of maternal cortisol reaches the fetus. Consequently, fetal glucocorticoid levels are lower than those in the mother.

The placenta also expresses the glucocorticoid receptor from an early stage of pregnancy, which suggests that glucocorticoids might have a role to play within the placenta itself. Indeed, cortisol has been shown to inhibit the proliferation of human villous and extravillous, trophoblast (Gennari-Moser et al. 2011) and to promote apoptosis in both rat (Waddell et al. 2000) and human placenta (Crocker et al. 2001). In the rat placenta, there is also evidence that glucocorticoids cause a reduction in vascularization. Likewise, altered placental vascular function is noted in pregnant women treated with glucocorticoids due to asthma (Clifton et al. 2001). These data, along with animal studies demonstrating that a reduction in placental 11β-HSD2 expression (with consequent glucocorticoid signaling) is associated with a decrease in placental glucose and amino acid transporters, are in keeping with the hypothesis that excess glucocorticoids have an adverse effect on fetal growth by influencing placental growth and function. It is therefore noteworthy that placental expression of 11β-HSD2 is reduced in association with FGR (McTernan et al. 2001) and that birthweight of individuals homozygous for mutations in the 11β-HSD2 gene are reduced in comparison to unaffected siblings (Dave-Sharma et al. 1998).

Although inhibition of 11β-HSD2 activity through maternal consumption of liquorice does not affect birthweight, their offspring exhibit numerous neurodevelopmental defects including impaired cognition and attention deficit (Raikkonen et al. 2009). In rats, 11β-HSD2 expression is decreased by maternal stress and it has been suggested that in humans also prenatal maternal anxiety/stress, including worries associated with pregnancy, adverse life events and even global events, such as terrorist attacks, influence neurodevelopment, especially in relation to affective behavior. Oxygen and maternal nutrition also regulate 11β-HSD2. Expression is decreased by hypoxia and in rodents, the activity of the enzyme is reduced by protein restriction; experiments using a placental cell line suggest that low levels of amino acids also cause decreased expression/activity in the human placenta.

Thyroid hormones

The thyroid hormones—thyroxine (T4) and triiodothyronine (T3)—are synthesized in and released from, the thyroid gland under the influence of thyroid stimulating hormone (TSH), which is produced in the anterior pituitary axis in response to the hypothalamic TSH releasing hormone (TRH). hCG has a similar structure to TSH and is able to activate the TSH receptor; consequently, levels of the maternal thyroid hormones are also regulated by this placental-derived biochemical. The thyroid hormones provide negative feedback to the hypothalamus and anterior pituitary to reduce TRH and TSH secretion.

Thyroid hormone synthesis depends on iodine, which is extracted from the circulation by the thyroid gland, oxidized to iodide and then added to specific tyrosine residues in a large glycoprotein known as thyroglobulin, to form monoiodtyrosine (MIT) or di-iodotyrosine (DIT). These are then coupled within thyroglobulin to generate T3 (one molecule of MIT coupled with one molecule of DIT) or T4 (two DIT molecules) and then the hormones are released from the thyroglobulin by proteolysis. The thyroid gland mainly secretes T4; T3 is largely produced by de-iodination of T4 in the periphery. T4 is converted to T3 through the action of the type I and type II deiodinases, which have differential tissue expression. The type III 3 deiodinase inactivates T4 by converting it to reverse T3 (rT3). The vast majority (99%) of thyroid hormones released into the circulation are bound by binding proteins, including thyroxine binding globulin (TBG), transthyretin and albumin, which serve as a circulating storage reservoir and to increase hormone half-life; they may also modulate hormone delivery to selected tissues.

Cellular uptake of the thyroid hormones is facilitated by several different families of membrane transporter molecules: monocarboxylate transporters (MCTs), system L amino acid transporters (LATs) and organic-anion-transporting polypeptides (OATPs). Inside the cell, the thyroid hormones mediate their effect by interacting with the thyroid receptor, which is a member of the steroid/thyroid hormone receptor superfamily. T3 has a greater affinity than T4 for the thyroid receptor and therefore, T3 is more biologically active.

During early pregnancy, there is a small increase in the maternal level of free T4, probably as a result of thyroid stimulation by hCG and consequent decrease in the circulating concentration of TSH. The maternal thyroid hormones can be taken up by the placenta as members of each of the families of transporters are expressed: MCT8, MCT10, LAT1, OATP1A2 and OATP4A1. It is thought that the thyroid hormones have a role within placenta as *in vitro*, cytotrophoblast proliferation, invasion (Oki et al. 2004, Barber et al. 2005) and differentiated function (hormone production) (Maruo et al. 1991) as all regulated by targets. As the fetus requires thyroid hormones for normal fetal growth and brain development, maternal thyroid hormones also cross the placenta, as evidenced by the detection of thyroid hormones in fetal tissues before the start of fetal thyroid gland function. Consequently in early pregnancy, the levels of circulating thyroid hormones in the fetus reflect those of the mother, albeit at lower concentrations. Interestingly, the concentration of T4 in the fetal CNS is also strongly correlated with maternal T4 levels (Dowling et al. 2000). The placenta must also transport iodine from mother to fetus to enable fetal production of thyroid hormones and it is speculated that it may store iodine as a mechanism for protecting the fetus from transient hypothyroidism due to fluctuations in maternal iodine intake and supply.

It is possible that the binding proteins transthyretin and albumin, which are produced by the placenta, are involved in transporting the thyroid hormones across the placenta to the fetal circulation, though they most likely have a role in modulating hormone access to deiodinases. Type II and type III deiodinanse, predominantly the latter, are expressed by the placenta, though their activity declines as gestation advances, which is thought to permit the increased fetal demand for thyroid hormones in later pregnancy.

Abnormalities in maternal thyroid function are common occurrences in pregnancy; both hyperthyroidism and hypothyroidism are associated with abnormal placental development resulting in pregnancy loss and complications such as FGR and pre-eclampsia (Negro and Mestman 2011). Autoimmune hypothyroid disease is responsible for most instances of hypothyroidism in the Western world, but globally iodine deficiency is the major cause of this condition (Negro and Mestman 2011).

Placentas from pregnancies complicated by FGR show altered expression of the thyroid transporters. MCT8 expression (Chan et al. 2006) and therefore T4 uptake is increased, but efflux is unaltered, resulting in an increase in placental trophoblast intracellular T3 concentrations (Vasilopoulou et al. 2010). There is also an increase in placental thyroid receptor expression (Kilby et al. 1998) and potentially sensitivity to T3, which is thought to contribute to the increase in trophoblast apoptosis observed in such placentas (Vasilopoulou et al. 2010). FGR is associated with low levels of thyroid hormones in cord blood (Kilby et al. 1998), suggesting reduced placental transfer.

Thyroid hormones are essential for normal brain development as they regulate neurogenesis, myelination, dendrite proliferation and synapse formation (Williams 2008); thus, all components of the thyroid hormone axis—transporter, type II deiodinase and the thyroid receptor, are present in the fetal brain from early in gestation. Consequently, abnormalities in maternal thyroid hormone levels are associated with impaired neural development in the offspring. Children of mothers with hypothyroidism score significantly lower than controls on IQ tests performed at ages 7–9 years (Haddow et al. 1999).

Conclusions

Brain development in utero is a highly sensitive process in which hormones from maternal and placental sources play important roles. In this complex system, a synergy of endocrine signaling is required throughout gestation, with different hormones impacting upon development in different ways, at different times. As summarized in Table 3.1, some, such as thyroid hormones and leptin, may cross the placenta to act directly on the developing nervous system, impacting on aspects of cellular function including neurogenesis, myelination and synapse formation. Others, including IGFs and pGH, operate indirectly to influence placental growth and therefore fetal development—including the CNS. Although the mechanisms for association between placental dysfunction, impaired fetal growth and neurodisability are still unclear, the relationships between endocrine output and neurological development, as outlined, suggest that hormonal influences from the placenta are vital for this process. In addition, appropriate regulation and signaling of these hormones are essential, as illustrated in instances of suboptimal environmental conditions, such as poor maternal dietary intake, which have implications for hormone expression, as well as genetic models in which altered receptor expression and therefore reduced signaling capacity also result in inadequate growth. Further studies, both clinical and *in vivo*, into the implications of disrupted hormone production in pregnancy and the subsequent impact on brain development and function would provide additional essential understanding as to the significance of these factors in this system.

TABLE 3.1
Consequences of altered maternal and placental hormone production/function on placental and fetal growth

Hormone	Can cross placenta to directly effect fetus	Consequence of altered expression/function	
hCG	Yes	↓	FGR
		↓ ↔	Pre-eclampsia
hCG-H		↓	Pre-eclampsia
Estrogen and progesterone	Yes	Therapeutic ↑	Treatment improves neurodevelopment in preterm, low-birthweight infants
Placental growth hormone	No	Early expression	Related to fetal growth rate
		↓ (term)	FGR
		GHR $^{-/-}$	Smaller placenta, low birthweight
Placental lactogen	Yes	↓ (term)	FGR
Insulin-like growth factors	Unknown	*In vivo* gene KOs:	Weight change:
		↓ IGF-I	40% fetal decrease, normal placenta
		↓ IGF-II	40% fetal, 25% placental decrease
		↓ IGF-I/IGF-II	60% fetal decrease, embryonic lethal
		↓ IGF1R	55% fetal decrease, normal placenta
		↓ IGF2R	40% fetal and placental increase
		↓ Placental specific IGF-II	25% fetal, 35% placental decrease
		Homozygous partial deletion IGF-I	Intrauterine and postnatal growth retardation
Leptin	Yes	Maternal obesity ↑	Leptin resistance in fetus; impaired fetal growth
		Leptin levels ↓ syncytial expression of receptor	↓ System A activity
		↓ levels umbilical vein	*In vivo* model of obesity- abnormal placental morphology and function, hypoxia in labyrinth
		↓ global levels (e.g., mutation)	FGR
			Delayed neurocognitive development (therapeutic administration improves)
Glucocorticoids 11ß-HSD2:	Yes	↑	Altered placental function
		Abnormal levels, for example, hypoxia, protein restriction	↓ placental glucose and amino acid transporters
		↓ levels	FGR
		↓ gene expression	Lower birthweight
		Inhibition	Impaired cognition and attention deficit
Thyroid hormones	Yes	Altered transporter expression	FGR
		↓ levels cord blood	FGR
		Altered receptor expression	FGR
		Hyperthyroidism and hypothyroidism common in pregnancy	Associated with pregnancy loss and other complications, for example, FGR and pre-eclampsia

FGR, fetal growth restriction; GHR, growth hormone receptor

REFERENCES

Ackerman GE, Carr BR (2002) Estrogens. *Rev Endocr Metab Disord* 3: 225.

Agodi A, Marranzano, M, Jones CS, Threlfall EJ (1995) Molecular characterization of trimethoprim resistance in salmonellas isolated in Sicily, 1985–1988. *Eur J Epidemiol* 11: 33.

al-Hader AA, Tao YX, Lei ZM, Rao CV (1997) Fetal rat brains contain luteinizing hormone/human chorionic gonadotropin receptors. *Early Pregnancy* 3: 323.

Albrecht ED, Bonagura TW, Burleigh DW, Enders AC, Aberdeen GW, Pepe GJ (2006) Suppression of extravillous trophoblast invasion of uterine spiral arteries by estrogen during early baboon pregnancy. *Placenta* 27(4–5), 483–490. doi: 10.1016/j.placenta.2005.04.005.

Bahado-Singh RO, Oz AU, Kingston JM, Shahabi S, Hsu CD, Cole L (2002) The role of hyperglycosylated hCG in trophoblast invasion and the prediction of subsequent pre-eclampsia. *Prenat Diagn* 22(6), 478–481. doi: 10.1002/pd.329.

Baker J, Liu JP, Robertson EJ, Efstratiadis A (1993) Role of insulin-like growth factors in embryonic and postnatal growth. *Cell* 75: 73.

Barber KJ, Franklyn JA, McCabe CJ et al. (2005) The *in vitro* effects of triiodothyronine on epidermal growth factor-induced trophoblast function. *J Clin Endocrinol Metab* 90(3), 1655–1661. doi: 10.1210/jc.2004-0785.

Beyer C (1999) Estrogen and the developing mammalian brain. *Anat Embryol (Berl)* 199: 379.

Bouret SG (2010) Neurodevelopmental actions of leptin. *Brain Res* 1350, 2–9. doi: 10.1016/j.brainres.2010.04.011.

Brelje TC, Scharp DW, Lacy PE et al. (1993) Effect of homologous placental lactogens, prolactins, and growth hormones on islet B-cell division and insulin secretion in rat, mouse, and human islets: Implication for placental lactogen regulation of islet function during pregnancy. *Endocrinology* 132(2), 879–889. doi: 10.1210/endo.132.2.8425500.

Catalano PM, Presley L, Minium J, Hauguel-de Mouzon S (2009) Fetuses of obese mothers develop insulin resistance in utero. *Diabetes Care* 32(6), 1076–1080. doi: 10.2337/dc08-2077.

Caufriez A, Frankenne F, Hennen G, Copinschi G (1993) Regulation of maternal IGF-I by placental GH in normal and abnormal human pregnancies. *Am J Physiol* 265: E572.

Chan S-Y, Franklyn JA, Pemberton HN et al. (2006) Monocarboxylate transporter 8 expression in the human placenta: The effects of severe intrauterine growth restriction. *J Endocrinol* 189, 465–471. doi: 10.1677/joe.1.06582.

Chard T (1994) Insulin-like growth factors and their binding proteins in normal and abnormal human fetal growth. *Growth Regul* 4: 91.

Chen JZJ, Sheehan PM, Brennecke SP, Keogh RJ (2012) Vessel remodelling, pregnancy hormones and extravillous trophoblast function. *Mol Cell Endocrinol* 349(2), 138–144. doi: 10.1016/j.mce.2011.10.014.

Chowen JA, Goya L, Ramos S et al. (2002) Effects of early undernutrition on the brain insulin-like growth factor-I system. *J Neuroendocrinol* 14: 163.

Christine KW (2008) Progesterone receptors and neural development: A gap between bench and bedside? *Endocrinology* 149(6), 2743–2749. doi: 10.1210/en.2008-0049.

Clifton VL, Giles WB, Smith R et al. (2001) Alterations of placental vascular function in asthmatic pregnancies. *Am J Respir Crit Care Med* 164(4), 546–553. doi: 10.1164/ajrccm.164.4.2009119.

Constância M, Hemberger M, Hughes J et al. (2002) Placental-specific IGF-II is a major modulator of placental and fetal growth. *Nature* 417, 945–948. doi: 10.1038/nature00819.

Crocker IP, Barratt S, Kaur M, Baker PN (2001) The in-vitro characterization of induced apoptosis in placental cytotrophoblasts and syncytiotrophoblasts. *Placenta* 22(10), 822–830. doi: 10.1053/plac.2001.0733.

Dave-Sharma S, Wilson RC, Harbison MD et al. (1998) Examination of genotype and phenotype relationships in 14 patients with apparent mineralocorticoid excess. *J Clin Endocrinol Metab* 83(7), 2244–2254. doi: 10.1210/jcem.83.7.4986.

Dechiara TM, Efstratiadis A, Robertsen EJ (1990) A growth-deficiency phenotype in heterozygous mice carrying an insulin-like growth factor II gene disrupted by targeting. *Nature* 345, 78–80. doi: 10.1038/345078a0.

Dos SC, Essioux L, Teinturier C, Tauber M, Goffin V, Bougneres P (2004) A common polymorphism of the growth hormone receptor is associated with increased responsiveness to growth hormone. *Nat Genet* 36: 720.

Dowling AL, Martz GU, Leonard JL, Zoeller RT (2000) Acute changes in maternal thyroid hormone induce rapid and transient changes in gene expression in fetal rat brain. *J Neurosci* 20: 2255.

Farley DM, Choi J, Dudley DJ et al. (2010) Placental amino acid transport and placental leptin resistance in pregnancies complicated by maternal obesity. *Placenta* 31(8), 718–724. doi: 10.1016/j. placenta.2010.06.006.

Forbes K, Westwood M (2008) The IGF axis and placental function: A mini review. *Horm Res* 69, 129–137. doi: 10.1159/000112585.

Forbes K, Westwood M, Baker PN, Aplin JD (2008) Insulin-like growth factor I and II regulate the life cycle of trophoblast in the developing human placenta. *Am J Physiol Cell Physiol* 294(6), C1313–C1322. doi: 10.1152/ajpcell.00035.2008.

Freemark M (2006) Regulation of maternal metabolism by pituitary and placental hormones: Roles in fetal development and metabolic programming. *Horm Res* 65, 41–49. doi: 10.1159/000091505.

French NP, Hagan R, Evans SF, Godfrey M, Newnham JP (1999) Repeated antenatal corticosteroids: Size at birth and subsequent development. *Am J Obstet Gynecol* 180(1 Pt 1): 114–121.

Gennari-Moser C, Khankin EV, Schüller S et al. (2011) Regulation of placental growth by aldosterone and cortisol. *Endocrinology* 152(1), 263–271. doi: 10.1210/en.2010-0525.

Gluckman PD, Hanson MA, Cooper C, Thornburg KL (2008) Effect of in utero and early-life conditions on adult health and disease. *N Engl J Med* 359, 61–73. doi: 10.1056/NEJMra0708473.

Godfrey K, Robinson S, Barker DJ, Osmond C, Cox V (1996) Maternal nutrition in early and late pregnancy in relation to placental and fetal growth. *BMJ* 312: 410.

González M, Cabrera-Socorro A, Pérez-García CG et al. (2007) Distribution patterns of estrogen receptor α and β in the human cortex and hippocampus during development and adulthood. *J Comp Neurol* 503(6), 790–802. doi: 10.1002/cne.21419.

Haddow JE, Palomaki GE, Allan WC et al. (1999) Maternal thyroid deficiency during pregnancy and subsequent neuropsychological development of the child. *N Engl J Med* 341: 549.

Han VK, Bassett N, Walton J, Challis JR (1996) The expression of Insulin-Like Growth Factor (IGF) and IGF-Binding Protein (IGFBP) genes in the human placenta and membranes: Evidence for IGF-IGFBP interactions at the feto-maternal interface. *J Clin Endocrinol Metab* 81(7), 2680–2693. doi: 10.1210/jcem.81.7.8675597.

Harris A, Seckl J (2011) Glucocorticoids, prenatal stress and the programming of disease. *Horm Behav* 59(3), 279–289. doi: 10.1016/j.yhbeh.2010.06.007.

Harris LK, Crocker IP, Baker PN, Aplin JD, Westwood M (2011) IGF2 actions on trophoblast in human placenta are regulated by the insulin-like growth factor 2 receptor, which can function as both a signaling and clearance receptor. *Biol Reprod* 84(3), 440–446. doi: 10.1095/biolreprod.110.088195.

Harris LK, Westwood M (2012) Biology and significance of signalling pathways activated by IGF-II. *Growth Factors*, 30(1), 1–12. doi: 10.3109/08977194.2011.640325.

Harvey J, Solovyova N, Irving A (2006) Leptin and its role in hippocampal synaptic plasticity. *Prog Lipid Res* 45(5), 369–378. doi: 10.1016/j.plipres.2006.03.001.

Hayes B, Sharif F (2009) Behavioural and emotional outcome of very low birth weight infants – literature review. *J Mater Fetal Neonatal Med* 22(10), 849–856. doi: 10.1080/14767050902994507.

Hedley P, Pihl K, Krebs L, Larsen T, Christiansen M (2009) Leptin in first trimester pregnancy serum: No reduction associated with small-for-gestational-age infants. *Reprod Biomed Online* 18: 832.

Henson MC, Castracane VD (2006) Leptin in pregnancy: An update. *Biol Reprod* 74(2), 218–229. doi: 10.1095/biolreprod.105.045120.

Kapoor A, Petropoulos S, Matthews SG (2008) Fetal programming of hypothalamic–pituitary–adrenal (HPA) axis function and behavior by synthetic glucocorticoids. *Brain Res Rev* 57(2), 586–595. doi: 10.1016/j.brainresrev.2007.06.013.

Kilby MD, Verhaeg J, Gittoes N, Somerset DA, Clark PMS, Franklyn JA (1998) Circulating thyroid hormone concentrations and placental thyroid hormone receptor expression in normal human pregnancy and pregnancy complicated by Intrauterine Growth Restriction (IUGR). *J Clin Endocrinol Metab* 83(8), 2964–2971. doi: 10.1210/jcem.83.8.5002.

Kirk SL, Samuelsson A-M, Argenton M et al. (2009) Maternal obesity induced by diet in rats permanently influences central processes regulating food intake in offspring. *PLoS ONE* 4(6), e5870. doi: 10.1371/journal.pone.0005870.

Klauwer D, Blum WF, Hanitsch S, Rascher W, Lee PD, Kiess W (1997) IGF-I, IGF-II, free IGF-I and IGFBP-1, -2 and -3 levels in venous cord blood: Relationship to birthweight, length and gestational age in healthy newborns. *Acta Paediatr* 86: 826.

Koutsaki M, Sifakis S, Zaravinos A, Koutroulakis D, Koukoura O, Spandidos DA (2011) Decreased placental expression of *hPGH, IGF-I* and *IGFBP-1* in pregnancies complicated by fetal growth restriction. *Growth Horm IGF Res* 21(1), 31–36. doi: 10.1016/j.ghir.2010.12.002.

Krantz D, Goetzl L, Simpson JL et al. (2004) Association of extreme first-trimester free human chorionic gonadotropin-β, pregnancy-associated plasma protein A, and nuchal translucency with intrauterine growth restriction and other adverse pregnancy outcomes. *Am J Obstet Gynecol* 191(4), 1452–1458. doi: 10.1016/j.ajog.2004.05.068.

Laviola L, Natalicchio A, Perrini S, Giorgino F (2008) Abnormalities of IGF-I signaling in the pathogenesis of diseases of the bone, brain, and fetoplacental unit in humans. *Am J Physiol Endocrinol Metab* 295(5), E991–E999. doi: 10.1152/ajpendo.90452.2008.

Lea RG, Howe D, Hannah LT, Bonneau O, Hunter L, Hoggard N (2000) Placental leptin in normal, diabetic and fetal growth-retarded pregnancies. *Mol Hum Reprod* 6: 763.

Louvi A, Accili D, Efstratiadis A (1997) Growth-promoting interaction of IGF-II with the insulin receptor during mouse embryonic development. *Dev Biol* 189(1), 33–48. doi: 10.1006/dbio.1997.8666.

Luo ZC, Nuyt AM, Delvin E et al. (2012) Maternal and fetal IGF-I and IGF-II levels, fetal growth, and gestational diabetes. *J Clin Endocrinol Metab* 97(5), 1720–1728. doi: 10.1210/jc.2011-3296.

Männik J, Vaas P, Rull K, Teesalu P, Rebane T, Laan M (2010) Differential expression profile of Growth Hormone/Chorionic Somatomammotropin genes in placenta of small- and large-for-gestational-age newborns. *J Clin Endocrinol Metab* 95(5), 2433–2442. doi: 10.1210/jc.2010-0023.

Maruo T, Matsuo H, Mochizuki M (1991) Thyroid hormone as a biological amplifier of differentiated trophoblast function in early pregnancy. *Acta Endocrinol (Copenh)* 125(1): 58–66.

Maymó JL, Pérez A, Gambino Y, Calvo JC, Sánchez-Margalet V, Varone CL (2011) Review: Leptin gene expression in the placenta – Regulation of a key hormone in trophoblast proliferation and survival. *Placenta* 32(Supplement 2), S146–S153. doi: 10.1016/j.placenta.2011.01.004.

McTernan CL, Draper N, Nicholson H et al. (2001) Reduced placental 11β-hydroxysteroid dehydrogenase Type 2 mRNA levels in human pregnancies complicated by intrauterine growth restriction: An analysis of possible mechanisms. *J Clin Endocrinol Metab* 86(10), 4979–4983. doi: 10.1210/jcem.86.10.7893.

Mise H, Yura S, Itoh H et al. (2007) The relationship between maternal plasma leptin levels and fetal growth restriction. *Endocr J* 54: 945.

Negro R, Mestman JH (2011) Thyroid disease in pregnancy. *Best Pract Res Clin Endocrinol Metab* 25(6), 927–943. doi: 10.1016/j.beem.2011.07.010.

Newbern D, Freemark M (2011) Placental hormones and the control of maternal metabolism and fetal growth. *Curr Opin Endocrinol Diabetes Obes* 18(6), 409–416. doi: 10.1097/MED.0b013e32834c800d.

Oki N, Matsuo H, Nakago S, Murakoshi H, Laoag-Fernandez JB, Maruo T (2004). Effects of 3,5,3′-triiodothyronine on the invasive potential and the expression of integrins and matrix metalloproteinases in cultured early placental extravillous trophoblasts. *J Clin Endocrinol Metab* 89(10), 5213–5221. doi: 10.1210/jc.2004-0352.

Paz-Filho G, Wong M-L, Licinio J (2011) Ten years of leptin replacement therapy. *Obes Rev* 12(5), e315–e323. doi: 10.1111/j.1467-789X.2010.00840.x.

Paz-Filho GJ, Babikian T, Asarnow R et al. (2008) Leptin replacement improves cognitive development. *PLoS ONE* 3(8), e3098. doi: 10.1371/journal.pone.0003098.

Pidoux G, Gerbaud P, Cocquebert M et al. (2012) Review: Human trophoblast fusion and differentiation: Lessons from trisomy 21 placenta. *Placenta* 33, Supplement, S81–S86. doi: 10.1016/j.placenta. 2011.11.007.

Räikkönen K, Pesonen AK, Heinonen K et al. (2009) Maternal licorice consumption and detrimental cognitive and psychiatric outcomes in children. *Am J Epidemiol* 170(9), 1137–1146. doi: 10.1093/aje/kwp272.

Rama S, Petrusz P, Rao AJ (2004) Hormonal regulation of human trophoblast differentiation: A possible role for 17β-estradiol and GnRH. *Mol Cell Endocrinol* 218(1–2), 79–94. doi: 10.1016/j.mce.2003.12.016.

Russo VC, Gluckman PD, Feldman EL, Werther GA (2005) The insulin-like growth factor system and its pleiotropic functions in brain. *Endocr Rev* 26(7), 916–943. doi: 10.1210/er.2004-0024.

Santos CD, Essioux L, Teinturier C, Tauber M, Goffin V, Bougnères P (2004) A common polymorphism of the growth hormone receptor is associated with increased responsiveness to growth hormone. *Nat Genet* 36, 720–724. doi: 10.1038/ng1379.

Schlotz W, Phillips DIW (2009) Fetal origins of mental health: Evidence and mechanisms. *Brain Behav Immun* 23(7), 905–916. doi: 10.1016/j.bbi.2009.02.001.

Sferruzzi-Perri AN, Owens JA, Standen P, Roberts CT (2008) Maternal insulin-like growth factor-II promotes placental functional development via the Type 2 IGF receptor in the guinea pig. *Placenta* 29(4), 347–355. doi: 10.1016/j.placenta.2008.01.009.

Shenkin SD, Starr JM, Deary IJ (2004) Birth weight and cognitive ability in childhood: A systematic review. *Psychol Bull* 130(6), 989–1013. doi: 10.1037/0033-2909.130.6.989.

Sooranna SR, Ward S, Bajoria R (2001a) Discordant fetal leptin levels in monochorionic twins with chronic midtrimester twin–twin transfusion syndrome. *Placenta* 22(5), 392–398. doi: 10.1053/plac.2001.0654.

Sooranna SR, Ward S, Bajoria R (2001b) Fetal leptin influences birth weight in twins with discordant growth. *Pediatr Res* 49, 667–672. doi: 10.1203/00006450-200105000-00010.

Stallings-Mann ML, Ludwiczak RL, Klinger KW, Rottman F (1996) Alternative splicing of exon 3 of the human growth hormone receptor is the result of an unusual genetic polymorphism. *Proc Natl Acad Sci U S A* 93: 12394.

Trotter A, Steinmacher J, Kron M, Pohlandt F (2012) Neurodevelopmental follow-up at five years corrected age of extremely low birth weight infants after postnatal replacement of 17β-estradiol and progesterone. *J Clin Endocrinol Metab* 97(3), 1041–1047. doi: 10.1210/jc.2011-2612.

Vasilopoulou E, Loubière LS, Martín-Santos A et al. (2010) Differential triiodothyronine responsiveness and transport by human cytotrophoblasts from normal and growth-restricted pregnancies. *J Clin Endocrinol Metab* 95(10), 4762–4770. doi: 10.1210/jc.2010-0354.

von Versen-Höynck F, Rajakumar A, Parrott MS, Powers RW (2009) Leptin affects system A amino acid transport activity in the human placenta: Evidence for STAT3 dependent mechanisms. *Placenta* 30(4), 361–367. doi: 10.1016/j.placenta.2009.01.004.

Waddell BJ, Hisheh S, Dharmarajan AM, Burton PJ (2000) Apoptosis in rat placenta is zone-dependent and stimulated by glucocorticoids. *Biol Reprod* 63: 1913.

Wagner CK (2008) Progesterone receptors and neural development: A gap between bench and bedside? *Endocrinology* 149: 2743.

Weinstock M (2005) The potential influence of maternal stress hormones on development and mental health of the offspring. *Brain Behav Immun* 19(4), 296–308. doi: 10.1016/j.bbi.2004.09.006.

Westwood M, Gibson JM, Sooranna SR, Ward S, Neilson JP, Bajoria R (2001) Genes or placenta asmodulator of fetal growth: Evidence from the insulin-like growth factor axis in twins with discordant growth. *Mol Hum Reprod* 7: 387.

Williams GR (2008) Neurodevelopmental and neurophysiological actions of thyroid hormone. *J Neuroendocrinol* 20(6), 784–794. doi: 10.1111/j.1365-2826.2008.01733.x.

Woods KA, Camacho-Hübner C, Savage MO, Clark AJL (1996) Intrauterine growth retardation and postnatal growth failure associated with deletion of the Insulin-Like Growth Factor I Gene. *N Engl J Med* 335, 1363–1367. doi: 10.1056/NEJM199610313351805.

Zygmunt M, Herr F, Keller-Schoenwetter S et al. (2002) Characterization of human chorionic gonadotropin as a novel angiogenic factor. *J Clin Endocrinol Metab* 87(11), 5290–5296. doi: 10.1210/jc.2002-020642.

4
THE RHEOLOGY OF UTERO-PLACENTAL AND FETO-PLACENTAL BLOOD FLOW

Ian Crocker

The juxtaposition between fetal and maternal circulations is arguably the most important feature of the human placenta, with aberrations on either side causal of fetal and maternal morbidity and mortality. With advancements in clinical imaging comes an expanded appreciation of the utero- and feto-placental vasculature, but the more subtle mechanistic adaptations which underpin these circulations are far from elucidated. This chapter highlights the major maternal and fetal vascular anatomical and rheological changes necessary for a successful pregnancy, but also uncovers misconceptions and knowledge gaps applicable to pathological pregnancies that may beget neurodevelopmental disorders.

The utero-placental vasculature
The architecture of the human uterine vasculature is well described (Fig. 4.1). Blood is delivered to the uterus via a dual arterial anastomotic loop from the ovarian arteries or uterine arteries, originating at the aorta and iliac arteries respectively. This bilateral anatomical arrangement provides the uterus with a dual supply of blood and the advantage of

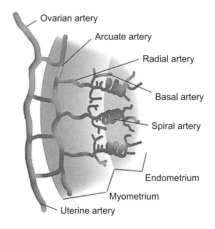

Fig. 4.1. The uterine blood supply, illustrating arterial arrangements within the main tissue zones.

redundancy in the case of interruption or occlusion. From these larger vessels, blood passes to the arcuate arteries within the myometrium, that encircle the organ. At this point, vessels from each side anastomose along the uterine midline. Smaller radial arteries emanate from these arcuate vessels and penetrate the myometrium. On passing through the myometrial–endometrial junction, these radial arteries split into smaller spiral arterioles that penetrate the endometrium and terminate close to the uterine lumen, in capillaries that in turn drain via venules into larger veins, eventually returning to the inferior vena cava.

Vascular preparation for implantation
In general, the basal endometrium and its vasculature remain relatively unchanged through-out the menstrual cycle. By contrast, its functional layers are constantly shifting in response to biochemical signals. The basal arteries are thought to be stable, non-hormone responsive structures, but the endometrial spiral arteries of the non-pregnant uterus show remarkable sensitivity to stimulation, typically from hormones (steroid and gonadotrophin) and angiogenic growth factors.

For embryo implantation to occur, the human endometrium must be singularly receptive. Studies in humans have demonstrated that endometrial blood flow rises during the proliferative phase of the menstrual cycle, peaking prior to ovulation. This rise in blood flow is largely maintained by vasodilatation and substantial increases in proliferation and angiogenesis, that is, the development of new capillaries from pre-existent vessels. Although circulating oestradiol positively correlates with endometrial blood flow, the mechanism is unclear, but is likely to favour nitric oxide stimulation. Our own data equally propose architectural changes to the tunica media, with a significant loss of smooth muscle arrangements (Fig. 4.2).

In general, oestradiol stimulates endometrial vascular permeability, while progesterone accelerates maturation of new vessels and exacerbates their dilatory capacity, up-regulating endothelial nitric oxide synthase (eNOS) expression. Within the oestrogen-primed endometrium, vascular endothelial growth factor (VEGF) intensifies vascular permeability,

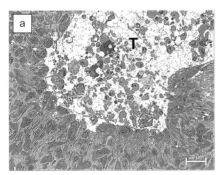 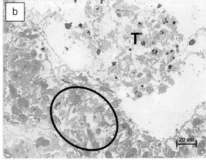

Fig. 4.2. Semi-thin tissue sections of myometrial microvessels perfused ex vivo with invasive placental trophoblast (T), (a) without and (b) with oestradiol co-treatment (10 nM). The oestrogen-exposed vessels show significant remodelling of the tunica media and mural smooth muscle (oval), which could facilitate further uterine vascular transformations.

endothelial cell proliferation and vessel formation. The angiopoietins, Ang-1 and Ang-2, fibroblast growth factor and platelet-derived growth factor have additional angiogenic responsibilities: Ang-1 destabilising vessels to initiate angiogenic growth and Ang-2 conferring stability on newly formed vessels. Neovascularisation, as opposed to angiogenesis, is also implicated. This more recently recognised form of de novo vessel formation is wholly reliant on endothelial progenitor cells and their sequestration from the maternal circulation. Oestradiol and VEGF are again primary regulators: oestradiol enhancing the numbers of endothelial progenitor cells and stimulating recruitment to the sites of vasculogenesis and VEGF mobilising bone-marrow-derived progenitor cells into the maternal uterine circulation.

Following implantation and endometrial decidualisation, vascularisation continues and growth factors increase proportionately. VEGF is exaggerated by human chorionic gonadotrophin and its receptor levels dictate embryo survival. At this stage, the importance of growth factors within this labile environment cannot be overstated. Disruptions to the balance of these angiogenic factors and their inhibitors are implicated in first-trimester miscarriage, while their disequilibrium can impose defective placentation, exacerbating the likelihood of utero-placental disorders of pregnancy.

Vessel transformations in the pregnant uterus
At week 2 of pregnancy, the invading human embryo is sustained by diffusion across a thin layer of vascular decidua, surrounding the syncytiotrophoblast mass. With growing metabolic demands, the implanted embryo requires direct contact with maternal blood. This is achieved by the physiological conversion of the maternal spiral arteries into highly dilated wide-mouthed sinusoids for high capacity, low resistance maternal flow. Although the extent of conversion varies across the placental bed, in general it extends through the decidua and into the inner third of the proximal myometrium. This process, which is considered fundamental for pregnancy success, is facilitated by a combination of placental-derived endovascular extravillous trophoblasts, which migrate down the spiral artery lumen and interstitial trophoblast cells, which invade through the endometrial stroma, subsequently penetrating the highly coiled vessels from outside in (Fig. 4.3a).

Although the molecular mechanisms orchestrating these vascular conversions are complex and unclear, the spiral arteries become stripped of their elastic lamina and vascular smooth muscle, rendering them unresponsive to vasomotor stimuli, creating highly dilated terminal coils of an anticipated 2–3mm in diameter. This transition ends abruptly at the endometrial–myometrial boundary, where the vascular lumen returns to its muscularised, unconverted size, some fourfold smaller than the spiral artery openings. Initially, trophoblast cells plug these unmodified regions, restricting access of maternal blood to the developing the placenta, but at around 10 weeks' gestation maternal blood flow ensues, flooding the intervillous space. At this point, the oxygen tension will rise dramatically, promoting vascular regression of peripheral villous capillaries and the generation of stem vessels to form lobular-like structures, ideally suited for nutrient and gaseous exchange.

In response to these changes and in contrast to other circulatory beds, the intervillous circulation of the human haemochorial placenta can be regarded as a more open system,

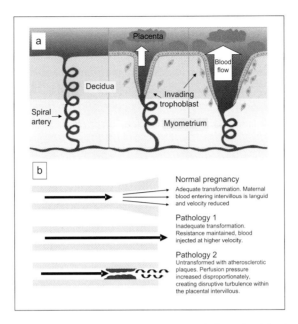

Fig. 4.3. Normal and abnormal transformations of uterine spiral arteries. The inadequate invasion/ activities of extravillous trophoblasts restrict luminal diameters and markedly attenuate intervillous blood flow (middle panel) (a) left-hand panel, pre-pregnancy; right-hand panel, pregnancy appropriate modifications. (b) The potential rheological consequences of insufficient artery transformations, including superimposed vasculopathy. Reproduced from *Placenta* 2007; 28, Supplement: S4–S13, with permission from Elsevier.

where spiral arteries discharge into the intervillous space, creating a lake of blood with little or no impedance to flow. In the rhesus monkey, where trophoblast invasion is restricted to the endometrium, spontaneous vasoconstriction of the myometrial spiral arteries accounts for intermittent intervillous flow during periods of constant maternal pressure. Although similar observations have been shown in humans during labour, the extent to which this occurs spontaneously is unclear, particularly in pathological pregnancies. From 2D Doppler quantification of pulsatile and non-pulsatile flow emanating from spiral arteries, jet-like streams of blood are reported at 20 weeks' gestation flooding the intervillous space, but thereafter non-pulsatile flow predominates (Collins et al. 2012). Although in this study, the number of pulsatile jets remaining at term was unrecorded, their pulsatility and resistance indexes in the third trimester were higher in pregnancies of small-for-gestational age infants. Notably, these differences were not emulated in the uterine arteries, as might be expected currently.

Uterine blood flow in early pregnancy

From weeks six to eight of gestation, profound changes occur in the maternal circulation, including a progressive increase in blood volume, increase in cardiac output and decrease in blood viscosity. To compensate, the dissociation curve for maternal oxyhaemoglobin shifts to the right and systemic resistance and pulmonary resistance are reduced, through hormonal and growth factor-mediated vasodilatation. In general, these haemodynamic adaptations, specifically those of the uterus, follow a continuum first established in the menstrual cycle, increasing uterine blood flow from 45 ml/min in the follicular phase to 750 ml/min at term. The significance of these pre-pregnancy adaptations is clearly evident in IVF-embryo transfer, where a transvaginal Doppler pulsatility index of between 2 and 3, as a measure of uterine artery blood velocity, indicates both optimal uterine receptivity and the likelihood of pregnancy success (Steer et al. 1995).

During pregnancy, the ultrasonographic assessment of the uterine artery is routinely favoured for scrutinising uterine blood flow. Nevertheless, its efficacy in monitoring downstream myometrial and decidual vessels is hotly debated. In addition to spiral artery conversions, these vessels undergo profound dilatation, particularly beneath the site of implantation, so much so that their diameter increases uniquely as they approach the placenta and even exceeds that of the uterine artery at term. In comparing Doppler measurements, a significant fall in impedance is noted within radial arteries midway through the first trimester, some 5 weeks prior to the uterine artery in the same pregnancy (Tamura et al. 2008). This lack of conformity holds equally for the physiological conversion of placenta-bed spiral arteries, which also fail to correlate universally with uterine artery waveforms. In explanation, it must be concluded that flow within spiral arteries and the placental intervillous space, has little impact on uterine resistance, questioning all previously held assumptions. In fact, discovered shunts within the myometrium, directly under the placental bed, imply that the bulk of flow passing through the uterine artery never reaches the endometrium at all (Schaaps et al. 2005). Conclusive evidence comes from Schaaps et al. (2005), who showed that uterine artery resistance remains unchanged even after placental delivery.

Along with these revelations comes a renewed requirement to reinterpret past and current Doppler assessments of utero-placental blood flow, especially those for the clinical prediction of adverse pregnancy outcomes. The current claim that uterine artery is a proxy for trophoblast remodelling of spiral arteries cannot be sustained and that the assertion that abnormal uterine artery Dopplers in the first trimester are directly associated with deficient trophoblast invasion must be re-evaluated. Insufficient remodelling of spiral arteries may indeed be present within these high-risk pregnancies and even indirectly related to sustained or raised uterine artery resistance. However, the true driving force for abnormal Doppler indexes is a lack of vascular conformity within the intact resistance vessels of the pregnant myometrial bed, that is, the radial and arcuate arteries. It is, therefore, tantalising to consider that this lack of vascular adaptation, specifically within the uterus, is the driving force behind many common placental-related obstetric complications, including fetal growth restriction (FGR) pre-eclampsia and pregnancy loss.

Endometrial denervation

Vasomotor tone and the modulation of vascular resistance within any vascular bed, including the uterus, are dependent upon extrinsic neural and humoral inputs, as well as intrinsic influences, such as myogenic regulation, flow and shear-induced vasodilation. Within the mammalian uterus, sympathetic innervation has high plasticity. In non-pregnant humans, the myometrial stroma has sparse nerve fibres, but a densely populated nerve plexus delineating the endometrial–myometrial interface. During pregnancy, a profound transient and reversible denervation of the uterus and uterine arteries occurs. This decrease in neural influence is concomitant with an elevation in myometrial smooth muscle and points to a sole dominance of non-neurogenic mechanisms for the regulation of uterine blood flow. The pathogenesis of reproductive loss is associated with uterine neural injuries pre-pregnancy, but paradoxically the retention of sympathetic control and thus its vaso-regulatory hold on blood vessels within the uterus, may also underpin some pregnancy complications. Although mostly conceptual, this idea is given credence from two studies highlighting greater abundance of nerve fibres in placenta-bed biopsies from women with pre-eclampsia (Quinn 2005, Fan et al. 2011). Although in both cases an association with unmodified spiral arteries was never established, nerves fibres were seen to accompany vessels of similar size within the decidua and myometrium (Fig. 4.4), suggesting neuronal-retained vascular control. Further work is undoubtedly necessary to confirm or refute these findings.

Intervillous blood flow

It is argued that haemodynamic adjustments, as a consequence of spiral artery conversions and other vascular adaptations, are crucial for the appropriate delivery of maternal blood across the relatively delicate villi of the human haemochorial placenta. As a defective trophoblast invasion and a failure to convert spiral arteries are associated with spontaneous miscarriage, FGR and early onset pre-eclampsia, it is highly plausible that these complications constitute a spectrum of disorders, varyingly attributable to early or late aberrations in the utero-placental circulation.

Given current limitations in imaging modalities, the evidence for and consequences of these uterine maladaptations is difficult to discern. Nevertheless, mathematical modelling, using literature-derived dimensions, has allowed appropriate and inappropriate utero-placental

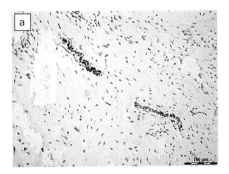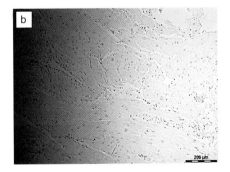

Fig. 4.4. Placental bed decidua and myometrium stained for large nerve fibres. (a) Samples from patients with preeclampsia show nerve fibres present (S100 stained). (b) Unaffected pregnancies show complete denervation. Reproduced from *Reprod Sci* 2011 18 (12): 1262–1266, with permission from SAGE Publications.

haemodynamics to be approximated and their consequences for human placental pathology explored (Burton et al. 2009). Within such models, adequate dilatation of the endometrial–myometrial arteries slows the rate of maternal blood flow from 2–3m/s to 10cm/s, with subsequent intervillous transit of 25–30s—a period for optimal exchange. In the absence of artery conversions, the same model predicts maternal blood will enter the intervillous space as turbulent jets of 1–2m/s with a diminished transit of 1s—a time wholly unfavourable for nutrient and gaseous delivery (Fig. 4.3b). Although partly offset by the intrauterine shunts, the increased momentum of these emerging jets may have profound damaging and remodelling effects on the labile placental villi and vasculature. One consequence, as noted by experienced sonographers, is the appearance of echogenic cystic (vascular) lesions, created by disruptions to villous branches. Within these areas, the centres of placental lobules become deeper and lined with thrombotic material. Continued exposure to these 'hose-like' spiral artery emissions forces the placenta lobule to become deeper, increasing maximum placental depth from 2–3cm to beyond 4cm, a now recognised predictor of placental pathology. In the most severe instances, more gross morphological changes can be identified sonographically through a 'jelly-like' or 'wobbly' placenta, in which anchoring placental villi are lost or disrupted (Toal et al. 2007). These placentas are seen to jerk under the force of entering blood. Such phenomena hold obvious clinical concerns and prompt obstetric scrutiny.

Within our laboratory studies, we have emulated these normal and abnormal intervillous flow patterns in an *ex vivo* dual perfused human placental model. In this system, a lobule of placenta, retained at delivery, is perfused with arterial and venous cannulation to replicate the fetal circulation and five separate cannulae, embedded within the maternal aspect, are used to emulate maternal spiral arteries. Using maternal perfusions of flow and pressure akin to those of normal pregnancy, villous integrity and transport activities are retained. However, under exaggerated and turbulent flow conditions, as espoused by the mathematical model, tissue disruption is recorded, as typified by syncytiotrophoblast shedding and oedema (Hutchinson et al. 2009). In these studies, liberated trophoblast fragments, collected under high velocity, turbulent conditions, showed stimulatory effects on exposed vascular endothelial and maternal inflammatory cells. These observations are in line with an excess of trophoblast material in placental pathologies, most notably pre-eclampsia and coincide with a maternal systemic response. Overall, these studies support the idea of a haemodynamic basis for placental-driven maternal morbidities, but further investigations are warranted.

Failure in the conversion of spiral arteries should not significantly limit the volume of maternal blood entering the placenta, but it has long been held that the pathological placenta is under-perfused and oxygen-deplete, that is, hypoxic. There is little evidence, metabolic or otherwise, to support this notion. An alternative prediction, with stronger support, is that the affected placenta is oxidatively stressed, most probably by ischaemia–reperfusion injury, through concomitant fluctuations in placenta oxygen (Burton and Jauniaux 2004). Within a unifying concept, the retention of smooth muscle around untransformed spiral arteries, perhaps with additionally retained nervation, increases the risk of spontaneous vasoconstriction in vessels, which would otherwise lack vasomotor control. Under these circumstances, rheological consequences for the utero-placenta predominate and damaging and inadequate intervillous flow transpires. Secondary and perhaps exacerbatory, would be acute atherosis and thrombosis, most notably within the radial or spiral arteries. These vascular deposits, typical of pre-eclampsia and pro-thrombotic conditions, could exacerbate the already disrupted blood flow within the intervillous placenta, markedly reducing the calibre of supplying vessels (Fig. 4.3b). In other vascular beds, these intra-luminal obstructions temporarily occlude arterioles, raising the chance of ischaemia–reperfusion. In the human placenta, villous infarction correlates nicely with decidual vasculopathy and evidence of both are cornerstones of placental pathology, as discussed throughout this book.

The feto-placental vasculature

HAEMODYNAMIC FORCES IN EMBRYONIC DEVELOPMENT

For over a century, it has been recognised that the physical forces imparted by blood flow play an important physiological role, none more so than in the developing yolk sac and embryo, where vasculogenesis and remodelling are crucial in early embryonic development. This influence is felt first in the yolk sac, where heartbeat and blood flow initiate the hierarchal remodelling of vessels of the primitive capillary plexus (for effective embryo perfusion) and subsequently in the embryo proper, where haemodynamic forces are responsible for developing the early vasculature, notably the heart, but also disparate developmental determinants, such as haematopoietic and neural divisions and stem cell differentiation and lineage commitments.

After initial phases of vascular remodelling, embryonic vessels undergo a process of stabilisation, largely mediated by endothelial and mural cell interactions. Again, haemodynamic forces play a significant role, strengthening these high-flow vessels and stimulating their maturation. The molecular basis of mechano-sensitivity which mediates this process is complex and ill-defined, but a variety of membrane-localised molecules, such as platelet endothelial cell adhesion molecule (PECAM-1), vascular endothelial growth factor 2 (VEGR2), vascular endothelial cell cadherin (VE-cadherin) and integrins, are implicated. These molecules detect either the circumferential stress, initiated by blood pressure, or frictional force or shear stress exerted by flow. Further components include ion channels, G-protein-coupled receptors, glycocalyx and mechano-sensory cilia, which protrude into the vessels and initiate the opening of calcium channels. The intracellular propagation of signals is better defined, through PI3K/AKT and MAPK pathways, while endothelial cells further communicate by paracrine means (as already specified in the uterus), or directly with smooth muscle through connecting porous membranes. In return, smooth muscle can modify endothelial gene expression, modulating responses to pressure and stress in the longer term, in essence re-programming vessels after reaching homeostasis.

Many breakthroughs in understanding the physiological role of haemodynamic force have been defined in embryogenesis, as similar effects are usually observed in the adult. As may be expected, dysfunctions in the mechano-sensory components of endothelial and smooth muscle cells have far reaching implications for pregnancy, exemplified in knockout mice, where resulting aberrations yield focal haemorrhage, cardiac dysmorphogenesis, growth retardation and eventual embryonic death. Given the lack of innervation of the human placenta, it could be assumed that these conserved responses have equal importance, instigating and directing vasculogenesis and remodelling throughout gestation. These mechanisms and their aberrations, could therefore be at the heart of some poorly defined feto-placental disorders; time and further research will tell.

VILLOUS PLACENTAL VASCULOGENESIS

The vascularisation of the human placenta is achieved de novo by the formation of vessels from mesenchymal precursor cells, as opposed to angiogenesis from pre-existing vessels. Within early placentation, fetal blood has yet to infiltrate the placental villous core but primitive vessels are formed from differentiating haemangioblasts, assisted by putative paracrine partners, such as Hofbauer cells and pericytes. Using knockout mice, it is clear that VEGR2 is crucial for the specification and early differentiation of these haemangioblasts and that VEGR1 orchestrates the early endothelial cells into tube-like structures (Fong et al. 1995, Shalaby et al. 1995). By week 4 of gestation, these rudimentary capillaries become connected to the developing umbilical cord, fetal heart and yolk sac vascular plexus. Although the heart is beating, an effective villous circulation is yet to be established. This delay is attributed to the dominance of nucleated erythrocytes and their lack of deformity. With their rapid decline, towards the end of the first trimester, a true feto-placental circulation begins. Evidence of mechano-regulation is suggested, as peri-vascular cell recruitment exclusively coincides with the onset of true fetal blood flow.

Once formed, the placental vascular network undergoes extensive and continual vasculogenic and angiogenic remodelling. These events have been reviewed extensively elsewhere, with the importance of VEGF, placental growth factor (PLGF), angiopoetins and oxygen repeatedly extolled. As a result, an extensive network develops, with the umbilical arteries dividing into first stem villous arteries and then branching into thin-walled intermediate villi, subsequently budding into abundant terminal villi and the sites of placental exchange. Throughout the first and second trimesters, there is a gradual increase in the number, volume and surface areas of capillaries within the villi, with their length accelerating exponentially from week 25 until term. On close inspection, it is clear that capillary diameters are not constant, particularly in terminal villi, where localised dilations, termed sinusoids, predominate, pushing the outer capillary wall into close association with the trophoblastic basement membrane. With subsequent thinning of the trophoblastic epithelium, it is considered that the pressure exerted by these distended capillaries creates specialised areas for diffusion. The importance of mechanical forces in sculpturing these regions is empathised by the fact that their thickness is directly related to the hydraulic pressures between the maternal and fetal circulations (Burton and Tham 1992). Although cyclic strains conceivably exist in these regions, shear stress is restricted to the larger muscularised stem and intermediate vessels. These vessels are therefore considered the major sites of placental vascular resistance.

DETERMINANTS OF PLACENTAL BLOOD FLOW

Umbilical blood flow increases throughout pregnancy, at term representing more than a fifth of fetal cardiac output. A direct estimation of flow is given by Doppler ultrasound, which although not readily quantifiable, provides a non-invasive insight into downstream placental resistance. The umbilical artery waveform in normal pregnancy indicates substantial flow in diastole. The absence or reversal of the end-diastolic component is highly indicative of increased resistance and strongly correlates with adverse pregnancy outcome, FGR and significant developmental sequelae (Alfirevic and Neilson 1995). Although this increased resistance may arise from inherent fetal abnormalities or reduced fetal cardiac output, in most instances the problem lies within the placenta itself, as a result of elaborations in local constrictors or structural alterations leading to impedance. In the umbilical veins, evidence of tightening of the umbilical ring at the level of the abdomen wall is also noted. The significance for fetal compromise remains unknown, but appropriate umbilical venous return could be of equal or greater importance than apposite passage through the placenta.

In general terms, placental blood flow is well preserved, even in the face of fetal adversity. In acute hypoxia, for example, blood is shunted away from the periphery towards the fetal heart, brain and placenta, thus maximising oxygen uptake and impact. In part, this is achieved through fetal synthesis of vasoconstrictors, preferentially constricting the peripheral circulation over that of the placenta, notable protagonists including catecholamines, angiotensin II, oxytocin and vasopressin. Within the placenta proper, low resistance predominates with global regulation restricted in favour of more localised paracrine activities. For vasoconstriction, thromboxane and endothelin-1 are implicated, especially in the umbilical circulation, while prostaglandins PGE2 and PGF, although stable, are far less potent. Vasodilatations may be initiated by prostacyclin I2, VEGF or PLGF, but the dominant force is shear stress through endothelial-induced nitric oxide production. In this context, a number of isoforms of nitric oxide synthase (NOS) are described in the placenta, even within the syncytiotrophoblast. Paradoxically, endothelial nitric oxide synthase (eNOS) expression is exaggerated in patients with placental compromise, explained as a compensatory response and local constrictions are also anticipated, with blood diverted to more functional regions of the placenta, akin to that of ventilation-flow matching in the lung.

Alterations in placental structure may contribute to an abnormal Doppler waveform and increased placental vascular resistance. Obvious causes are areas of infarction, microthrombus and other pathological lesions, but more subtle changes can also occur, such as altered numbers, aberrations and changes in calibre of vessels. In assessing the impact of these changes on Doppler flow, computer modelling of the feto-placental circulation has proven useful. Remarkably, such a model predicts that 50% obliteration of the small placental arteries is necessary before the Doppler pulsatility index will rise significantly (Thompson and Trudinger 1990). This finding nicely illustrates the reserve capacity of the human placenta. In assessing more subtle anomalies, both vascular casts and stereology have been applied to pregnancies of growth restriction and aberrant umbilical artery waveforms (Krebs et al. 1996, Mayhew et al. 2003). In general, terminal capillary loops appear sparse, longer and less branched than those of normal pregnancy and avascular regions are noted. Although the precipitating cause of these malformations is unclear, it is postulated that these changes will reduce oxygen extraction, hampering further placental and fetal development. Regardless, vascular resistance is undeniably linked to the structure of the human placenta and this feature, singularly or in addition to alterations in dilatation or function, has a direct impact on fetal well-being.

Conclusion

The importance and interplay between utero-placental and feto-placental blood flow in determining fetal development is difficult to discern. Current methods for accessing flow patterns in the most crucial compartments of the human placenta are wanting. In their absence, routine clinical assessments, typically ultrasound, rely solely on upstream and downstream surrogates, creating numerous misconceptions. Despite their crude nature, these tools frequently correlate with poor pregnancy outcome and fetal compromise and thus retain their clinical advantage. From current knowledge, it appears that the human placenta is generally well equipped to cope with most acute and minor haematologic disturbances, adapting locally to changes in supply and demand. It would therefore appear that only when more sustained and exaggerated challenges occur, or when these placental compensatory mechanisms falter, do chances of in utero complications and perinatal and neonatal sequelae arise.

REFERENCES

Alfirevic Z, Neilson JP (1995) Doppler ultrasonography in high-risk pregnancies: Systematic review with meta-analysis. *Am J Obstet Gynecol* 172(5): 1379–1387. doi: 10.1016/0002-9378(95)90466-2.

Burton GJ, Jauniaux E (2004) Placental oxidative stress: From miscarriage to preeclampsia. *Reprod Sci* 11(6): 342–352. doi 10.1016/j.jsgi.2004.03.003.

Burton GJ, Tham SW (1992) Formation of vasculo-syncytial membranes in the human placenta. *J Dev Physiol* 18(1): 43–47.

Burton GJ, Woods AW, Jauniaux E, Kingdom JCP (2009) Rheological and physiological consequences of conversion of the maternal spiral arteries for uteroplacental blood flow during human pregnancy. *Placenta* 30(6): 473–482. doi 10.1016/j.placenta.2009.02.009.

Collins SL, Birks JS, Stevenson GN et al. (2012) Measurement of spiral artery jets: General principles and differences observed in small-for-gestational-age pregnancies. *Ultrasound Obstet Gynecol* 40(2): 171–178. doi: 10.1002/uog.10149.

Crocker I (2007) Gabor than award lecture 2006: Pre-eclampsia and villous trophoblast turnover: Perspectives and possibilities. *Placenta*: 28: S4–S13. doi: 10.1016/j.placenta.2007.01.016.

Fan R, Qiu L, Huang X et al. (2011) Increased nerve fibers in placental bed myometrium in women with preeclampsia. *Reprod Sci* 18(12): 1262–1266. doi: 10.1177/1933719111411730.

Fong GH, Rossant J, Gertsenstein M, Breitman ML (1995) Role of the Flt-1 receptor tyrosine kinase in regulating the assembly of vascular endothelium. *Nature* 376: 66–70. doi:10.1038/376066a0.

Hutchinson ES, Brownbill P, Jones NW et al. (2009) Utero-placental haemodynamics in the pathogenesis of pre-eclampsia. *Placenta* 30(7): 634–641. doi: 10.1016/j.placenta.2009.04.011.

Krebs C, Macara LM, Leiser R et al. (1996) Intrauterine growth restriction with absent end-diastolic flow velocity in the umbilical artery is associated with maldevelopment of the placental terminal villous tree. *Am J Obstet Gynecol* 175(6): 1534–1542. doi: 10.1016/S0002-9378(96)70103-5.

Mayhewf TM, Ohadike C, Baker PN et al. (2003) Stereological investigation of placental morphology in pregnancies complicated by pre-eclampsia with and without intrauterine growth restriction. *Placenta* 24(2–3): 219–226. doi: 10.1053/plac.2002.0900.

Quinn M (2005)Pre-eclampsia and partial uterine denervation. *Med Hypotheses* 64(3): 449–454. doi: 10.1016/j.mehy.2004.08.027.

Schaaps JP, Tsatsaris V, Goffin F et al. (2005) Shunting the intervillous space: New concepts in human uteroplacental vascularisation. *Am J Obstet Gynecol* 192(1): 323–332. doi: 10.1016/j.ajog.2004.06.066.

Shalaby F, Rossant J, Yamaguchi TP et al. (1995) Failure of blood-island formation and vasculogenesis in Flk-1-deficient mice. *Nature* 376: 62–66. doi: 10.1038/376062a0.

Steer CV, Tan SL, Dillon D, Mason BA, Campbell S (1995) Vaginal color Doppler assessment of uterine artery impedance correlates with immunohistochemical markers of endometrial receptivity required for the implantation of an embryo. *Fertil Steril* 63(1): 101–108.

Tamura H, Miwa I, Taniguchi K et al. (2008) Different changes in resistance index between uterine artery and uterine radial artery during early pregnancy. *Hum Reprod* 23(2): 285–289. doi: 10.1093/humrep/dem375.

Thompson RS, Trudinger BJ (1990) Doppler waveform pulsatility index and resistance, pressure and flow in the umbilical placental circulation: An investigation using a mathematical model. *Ultrasound Med Biol* 16(5): 449–458. doi: 10.1016/0301-5629(90)90167-b.

Toal M, Chan C, Fallah S et al. (2007) Usefulness of a placental profile in high-risk pregnancies. *Am J Obstet Gynecol* 196(4): 363.e1– 363.e7. doi: 10.1016/j.ajog.2006.10.897.

5
INFLAMMATION AND PLACENTATION

Karen Racicot and Gil Mor

Immunology of pregnancy

Over 50 years ago, the renowned transplant immunologist, Sir Peter Medawar, proposed a theory as to why the fetus, a semi-allograft, is not rejected by the maternal immune system. He recognised for the first time the unique immunology of the maternal–fetal interface and its potential relevance for transplantation. In his original work, he described the 'fetal allograft analogy' where the fetus is viewed as a semi-allogeneic conceptus (made of paternal antigens and therefore foreign to the maternal immune system) which, by unknown mechanisms, evades rejection by the maternal immune system (Medawar 1948, Billingham et al. 1953). Subsequent studies demonstrated the presence of an active maternal immune system at the implantation site, providing evidence to support Medawar's original notion. As a result, investigators began to pursue the mechanisms by which the fetus escapes such maternal immune surveillance. Since Medawar's original observation, numerous studies have been performed in order to explain this paradigm, many of which have been centred on how the fetus and placenta fight against an active and aggressive maternal immune system. With placental trophoblast cells interacting directly with the mother's uterine cells, Colbern and Main eventually redefined the conceptual framework of reproductive immunology, as one of maternal–placental tolerance rather maternal–fetal tolerance, thus focusing attention on the interaction of the maternal immune system to the placenta and not the fetus (Colbern and Main 1991).

Inflammation and pregnancy

For many years, pregnancy was characterised as an anti-inflammatory condition and a shift in the type of cytokines produced would lead to abortion or pregnancy complications (Wegmann and Guilbert 1992). Although this theory was embraced enthusiastically and supported by many, an equal number of studies have argued against this notion (Chaouat et al. 1997, Ng et al. 2002, Saito et al. 2006). Reasons for these contradictions may be oversimplification of disparate observations during pregnancy. In general, pregnancy was evaluated as a single event, when in reality it has three distinct immunological phases, characterised by distinct biological processes (Mor and Cardenas 2010, Mor et al. 2011): implantation, placentation and parturition.

Implantation and early placentation, which occurs during the first and early second trimesters, resemble 'an open wound', one that requires a strong inflammatory response. Recent data, from our laboratory and others, indicate that inflammation is a critical step for preparing the epithelium of the uterus to become receptive to the embryo. Soluble factors, mainly cytokines and chemokines, secreted by dendritic cells induce the local degradation of mucin 1 (MUC1) that prevents the attachment of the highly adhesive blastocyst to an improper site (Gnainsky et al. 2010). Moreover, dendritic cells factors enhance the expression of adhesion molecules on the surface of the epithelium, allowing blastocyst attachment (Holmberg et al. 2012, Plaks et al. 2008). Following attachment, the embryo has to (1) break through the epithelial lining of the uterus in order to implant, (2) damage the endometrial tissue to invade and (3) replace the endothelium and vascular smooth muscle of the maternal blood vessels in order to secure an adequate blood supply. All these activities create a veritable 'battleground' of invading cells, dying cells and repairing cells, with an inflammatory environment required in order to secure the adequate repair of the uterine epithelium and removal of cellular debris to prevent the 'leak' of implanting/paternal antigens that could induce an immune response. Thus, the first trimester of pregnancy is a pro-inflammatory phase.

The second immunological phase of pregnancy is, in many ways, the optimal time for the mother. This is a period of rapid fetal growth and development. The mother, placenta and fetus are symbiotic and the predominant immunological feature is induction of an anti-inflammatory state. During the last immunological phase of pregnancy, the fetus has completed its development; all the organs are functional and parturition can only be achieved through renewed inflammation. This is characterised by an influx of immune cells into the myometrium in order to promote recrudescence of an inflammatory process. This pro-inflammatory environment promotes the contraction of the uterus, expulsion of the fetus and rejection of the placenta. Consequently, healthy pregnancy is both a pro-inflammatory and anti-inflammatory state, depending on time of gestation (Mor and Cardenas 2010, Racicot et al. 2014).

Unfortunately, the same cells that support a successful pregnancy can also be activated or stimulated to become detrimental to pregnancy. Intrauterine microbial invasion, resulting in an acute inflammation, characterised by infiltration of immune cells and secretion of inflammatory cytokines, is a potential major contributor to fetal injury and preterm birth (Koga et al. 2009). When microbial or danger signals are detected in the intrauterine cavity, the inflammatory response is initiated by innate immune receptors, the pattern recognition receptors (Abrahams et al. 2008). This is followed by secretion of cytokines that can cause direct damage to the placenta and/or promote activation of immune cells, causing them to shift away from a tolerogenic phenotype. Consequently, inflammation is necessary for healthy pregnancy, but pathological inflammation at the placenta may also result in complications which compromise the fetus, its resilience and normal development.

Inflammation and implantation
As the blastocyst travels from the fallopian tube to the uterine cavity, the surface epithelium of the uterus functions as the first contact responsible for adequate attachment of the trophoectoderm to the epithelium and subsequent trophoblast invasion and placentation. When a mammalian blastocyst enters the uterine cavity, the surface epithelium of the uterus is covered by molecules, such as MUC1 or MUC16 carbohydrates, that prevent the attachment of the blastocyst to an improper site. Indeed, in the human endometrium MUC1 and MUC16 are upregulated during the implantation 'window' (Meseguer et al. 2001, Simon et al. 2000). This suggests that the human endometrial surface epithelium prevents blastocyst adhesion, except for the precise

spot where the embryo attaches. In recent studies, we have shown that cytokines/chemokines produced by dendritic cells/macrophages in the uterine stroma induce local degradation of MUC1 and MUC16, which enable blastocyst attachment (Plaks et al. 2006, 2008, Holmberg et al. 2012). In addition, these cytokines/chemokines can enhance the expression of adhesion molecules necessary for these trophoblast-endometrium interactions (Gnainsky et al. 2010).

There are four ways by which the binding of the blastocyst to the epithelium may be enhanced: (1) stored adhesion molecules can be rapidly moved to the cell surface, (2) through inflammation-induced expression of new adhesion molecules, (3) by increased affinity of specific molecules following initial cell contact and (4) by reorganisation of adhesion molecules on the epithelial surface. Either of these possibilities or a combination can represent the response of the endometrial epithelium to DCs recruited to the site of implantation.

Role of immune cells and secreted factors

There are two major populations of immune cells within in the decidua: uterine natural killer (uNK) cells (70%) and macrophages (10%–30%). However, DCs (2%–5%) and populations of T and B-lymphocytes are also reported (1%–5%). These immune cells have a unique phenotype within the decidua and actively contribute to the tolerance of the embryo/fetus and placenta. It is widely considered that a shift in these cells to an activated inflammatory phenotype, due to infection, injury or misregulation of immunomodulatory factors, instigates a less tolerogenic environment, with the potential for fetal injury or demise.

UTERINE NATURAL KILLER CELLS

The largest population of immune cells in the decidua are uterine natural killer (uNK) cells. It is becoming increasingly clear that this cell type plays a crucial role in species with invasive placentation. In humans, these cells represent approximately 70% of the total leukocyte population and are characterised by surface markers, CD56[bright] and CD16[-] NK cells (Hanna et al. 2006, Moffett and Loke 2006). In normal pregnancy, there is evidence that these cells regulate spiral artery formation and control the invasion of trophoblast into the endometrium, probably by secreting pregnancy-promoting cytokines (Moffett and Loke 2006, Manaster and Mandelboim 2008). Interestingly, these cells are highly cytotoxic when activated in other tissues and circulation; therefore, it is important that factors remain present to maintain their tolerogenic phenotype (Hanna et al. 2006, Manaster and Mandelboim 2010). One important cytokine that promotes this in pregnancy is interleukin (IL)-10. Although the mechanism remains obscure, there is evidence which supports IL-10 as major suppressor of uNK cytotoxicity. In mice lacking this cytokine, very low doses of lipopolysaccharide (LPS) induce an inflammatory response and uNK activation, resulting in fetal loss (Murphy et al. 2005). Notably, some patients with unexplained spontaneous abortion have lower concentrations of this cytokine (Plevyak et al. 2002), supporting this IL-10/uNK rheostat in controlling excessive inflammation.

UTERINE DENDRITIC CELLS

Dendritic cells are professional antigen-presenting cells, able to elicit cytotoxic or tolerant phenotypes from adaptive immune cells. Within the decidua, these uterine dendritic cells (uDCs) infiltrate and participate in cross-talk with uNK cells (Blois et al. 2008), helping to maintain pregnancy by down-regulating uNK activation receptors and secreting the aforementioned, IL-10. Studies have shown that depletion of uDCs results in a severe impairment of implantation and embryo resorption in mice (Plaks et al. 2008). These experiments indicated that uDCs alone do not influence tolerance, but rather decidualisation. In agreement, we have shown that therapy with DCs in mice significantly decreased spontaneous resorption rates (Laskarin et al. 2007, Mor et al. 2011). Combined, these data propose a complementary involvement of uDCs in the pregnancy immune response, including a trophic role in the regulation of implantation.

Uterine macrophages

Macrophages are the predominant subset of human leukocyte antigen-presenting cells within the human decidua, comprising 20%–25% of all decidual leukocytes (Nagamatsu and Schust 2010). Their main markers are CD14+, HLA-DR+ and CD68+. These macrophages exhibit high levels of phenotypic plasticity and participate in diverse physiologic processes during pregnancy, adapting through marker expression and cytokine production to the local microenvironment. Accumulative evidence suggests involvement of uterine macrophages in a wide range of gestational processes including implantation, placental development and cervical ripening (Abrahams et al. 2004, Mor et al. 2006, Nagamatsu and Schust 2010).

In general, decidua macrophages present a phenotype related to tissue renewal and repair, also known as M2 macrophages (Mills et al. 2000). There are at least two major macrophage sub-types: M1 and M2 (Mantovani et al. 1992). M1 macrophages are under the influence of pro-inflammatory cytokines and secrete tumour necrosis factor (TNF) and IL-12 and participate in inflammation in response to micro-organisms. M2 polarisation is characterised by enhanced expression of scavenger receptors, mannose receptors, secretion of IL-1 receptor antagonist and a reduction in IL-12 expression (Mantovani et al. 2005). These M2 properties support the role of decidua macrophages in tissue renewal and inflammatory suppression during trophoblast invasion and placental growth.

An appropriate 'clean-up' of dying trophoblast prevents the release of paternal antigens that could trigger a maternal immune response against the fetus (Abraham et al. 2004). On the other hand, several aspects of parturition, including cervical ripening, the onset of labour and post-partum repair of the uterine cervix, are associated with pro-inflammatory macrophage activity and an M1-type prominence (Mackler et al. 1999, Young et al. 2002, Sakamoto et al. 2005). This plasticity of decidual macrophages to the micro-environment is deemed critical for normal pregnancy, with impairments in function linked to pathophysiology of abnormal gestations, including preterm labour and pre-eclampsia (Mor et al. 2006, Nagamatsu and Schust 2010). Although our understanding has increased significantly with regard to uterine macrophages, further research is required to identify signals that ultimately control their differentiation/activation within the human decidua.

Lymphocytes: T-regulatory cells

CD4+/CD25+ regulatory T cells (Tregs) were first described as a sub-population of T cells responsible for the maintenance of immunological self-tolerance by actively suppressing self-reactive lymphocytes (Sakaguchi et al. 1995). In the same way, these cells play a central role preventing autoimmunity, it is thought that Tregs are critical in preventing an immunological response to fetal antigens released during pregnancy (Somerset et al. 2004, Leber et al. 2010). During human pregnancy, a systemic expansion of Tregs is observed from early stages (Mjosberg et al. 2010). Evidence suggests Tregs are specific to paternal-derived cells, indicating a protective role for fetal cells (Jasper et al. 2006). Some infertility has been linked to the reduced expression of the Treg transcription factor Foxp3 in endometrial tissue. Similarly, spontaneous abortion correlates with lower systemic Treg levels, as compared to uncomplicated pregnancies (Sasaki et al. 2004, Zenclussen et al. 2005).

Although widely studied, factors behind Treg cell expansion in pregnancy remain ill-defined. It is proposed that hormonal changes may be involved, independent of paternal antigens, or that paternal antigens are required, with conceivable expansion as early as the time of insemination (Arruvito et al. 2007, Schumacher et al. 2007). In vitro, factors released by trophoblast cells induce CD4$^+$T cell differentiation into Tregs (Ramhorst et al. 2012). Although numerous questions remain, particularly regarding their regulatory mechanisms and origins, it is clear that Tregs play a central role in determining the maternal immune response to the placenta.

T helper-1/T helper-2 balance of pregnancy
Immune cells mediate their effects through cytokine release and secreted factors, to establish a desired micro-environment. In other words, immune cells, through cytokine production, create either a pro- or anti-inflammatory setting (Saito 2000, Saito et al. 2006). The cytokine profile created by immune cells can shape the characteristics of subsequent immune responses. For example, naïve T helper lymphocytes (Th-0) originate in the thymus and play a major role in creating specific micro-environments within the periphery, depending upon their differentiation status. If a Th-0 cell differentiates into a Th-1 cell, it secretes interleukin-2 (IL-2) and interferon-γ (IFN-γ), setting the basis for a cellular, cytotoxic immune response. Conversely, differentiation to a Th-2 subtype promotes secretion of cytokines, such as IL-4, IL-6 and IL-10, which are predominately involved in antibody production (Saito 2000, Saito et al. 2006). Therefore, cytokine micro-environments can be broadly grouped into two major categories: pro-inflammatory Th1, and anti-inflammatory Th2.

Although Th-1 and Th-2 are named after the types of T-lymphocytes that secrete these cytokines, this terminology is misleading, as several cell types are responsible for the secretion of these factors especially within the decidua and placenta. For many years, pregnancy was associated with a Th-2 phenotype, which was thought to suppress leucocytes and support immune tolerance. Although this is partly correct, as discussed above, it is now clear that during the early first trimester and late third trimester, inflammation is required for implantation and parturition respectively. Specifically, an inflammatory Th-1 environment is needed to secure the adequate attachment of the blastocyst to the uterine epithelium, repair of the epithelium and the removal of cellular debris during implantation and invasion of the trophectoderm (Dekel et al. 2010, Mor et al. 2006, 2011), and likewise, Th-1 must predominate once the fetus has completed development, when parturition is achieved through renewed inflammation. Between these times, the uterus maintains a Th-2 environment and a symbiotic, anti-inflammatory state between mother, placenta and fetus, in support of rapid fetal growth and development (Mor and Cardenas 2010, Mor et al. 2011).

Infection and inflammation in pregnancy

As further outlined in the next chapter, bacterial and viral infections pose a significant threat to pregnancy and fetal well-being, by gaining access to gestational tissues, such as decidua, placenta or fetal membranes, through one of three major routes: (1) ascending into the uterus from the lower tract, (2) descending into the uterus from the peritoneal cavity or (3) via the maternal circulation. There are strong clinical links between bacterial infection and preterm labour. Indeed, infections are reportedly responsible for up to 40% of preterm labours (Romero et al. 2002, Kim et al. 2004, Espinoza et al. 2006, Arechavaleta-Velasco et al. 2008, Madsen-Bouterse et al. 2010). While less is known about the impact of viruses on pregnancy outcome (Cardenas et al. 2010), their role in pregnancy complications is increasingly realised from clinical and experimental studies. As now discussed, infections that do not result in obvious obstetric issues still hold potential to infect the fetus or disrupt the feto-placental micro-environment, resulting in neonatal and developmental sequelae (Fig. 5.1) (Cardenas et al. 2010).

Inflammation on neuronal development

'The stage must be set before the play begins' is a perfect analogy for the relationship between the placenta and developing fetus. A 'genetically healthy fetus' will only become a healthy neonate with a well-developed placenta, provided with adequate nutrients, devoid

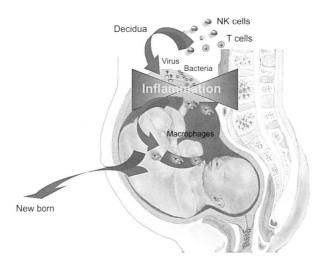

Fig. 5.1. Model of maternal–fetal interactions: The maternal and fetal immune systems maintain a continued interaction during pregnancy keeping a delicate balance that protects the fetus and mother. Viral infection of the placenta/decidua unit may alter this communication leading to dangerous signals and inflammation that affects the function of the maternal immune system and consequently leads to a detrimental impact on fetal development.

of environmental challenges, including, but certainly not limited to, infection and inflammation. The influence of the in utero environment on the developing fetus has been a topic of study for several decades, with the notion of developmental plasticity, or the ability of environmental factors to influence fetal development, first realised by David Barker and associates in the 1980s (Barker 1994). In pivotal epidemiological studies of women in England, they discovered a correlation between low birthweight and adult coronary heart disease, observations which highlighted the vulnerability of the fetus in utero. Ever since, multitudes of epidemiological studies have extended this hypothesis to other adult diseases, and recent clinical and animal trials have sort to understand this 'programming' phenomenon.

EPIDEMIOLOGICAL AND CORRELATIVE STUDIES

Epidemiological studies first showed a correlation between infection in pregnancy (bacterial and viral) and neurodevelopmental disorders in offspring. Likewise, maternal inflammation has been linked to the development of schizophrenia, autism, psychosis and related juvenile and adult disorders (Buka et al. 2001, Patterson 2009). It was subsequently proposed that infection led to an induction of pro-inflammatory cytokines, disrupting or altering fetal brain development (Gilmore and Jarskog 1997). Since then, prospective cohort studies have further defined the role physiological and pathophysiological maternal cytokines in the development of the fetal brain and central nervous system. For example, Brown and colleagues demonstrated that schizophrenia was associated with elevated concentrations of maternal IL-8 and serological evidence of influenza during pregnancy (Brown et al. 2004), while Buka and associates showed that maternal TNF-alpha concentrations, during late pregnancy, were correlated with development of psychosis in offspring (Buka et al. 2001). It is of note also that TNF-alpha is elevated in the cerebrospinal fluid of children with autism (Chez et al. 2007) and that neuro-inflammation, defined by MCP-1 in the brain and CSF, alongside immune-cytochemical evidence of microglia activation, are present in patients with autism of all ages (Vargas et al. 2005).

EXPERIMENTAL ANIMAL MODELS

Numerous animal studies have been utilised to better understand the mechanisms of maternal infection and inflammation resulting in aberrant neurological development and psychological abnormalities. Animal models, including rodents, rabbits and sheep, have been injected with toll-like receptors (TLR) ligands to determine if inflammation, downstream of TLR signalling, has effects on the development of offspring or their behaviour. In such studies, both LPS (ligand for TLR4) and Poly (I:C) (ligand for TLR3) during pregnancy lead to defects in prepulse inhibition, social interactions and learning potential of offspring (Patterson 2009). Upon further evaluation, these animals exhibited brain inflammation and altered microglia, suggesting that TLRs induced a response that causes deviations in the brains of these animals, preceding developmental and behavioural problems in later life. Similar observations were made when animals were infected with influenza and indeed, poly (I:C) or virus-treated animals had comparable cerebellar pathology to that of humans with autism (Patterson 2009, Shi et al. 2009).

Using a rodent model of maternal immune activation, a very elegant study has described (at least in part) the mechanism of how virally induced IL-6 can impact upon brain development (Smith et al. 2007). In this study, it was shown that a single injection of IL-6 had similar effects on prepulse inhibition as poly (I:C), with latent inhibition in the offspring. Neutralising IL-6 antibody injections, in conjunction with poly (I:C), prevented both these behavioural defects and irregular gene expression. Our own studies, using MHV-68 infection, have shown that infection of the placenta and subsequent inflammation have detrimental effects on fetal brain anatomy, characterised by changes in vascularity, leading to hydrocephalus, defined as an increase in the subarachnoid space (Cardenas et al. 2009). Studies like these are improving our understanding of how inflammation can lead to latent debilitating neurological disorders in humans.

Conclusion

The maternal immune system plays a central role in the development of normal pregnancy. From early implantation to parturition, each immune cell type contributes to a specific developmental phase, creating a unique environment to orchestrate cell and tissue function. Similarly, during each phase of pregnancy the immune system helps to create a unique cytokine/chemokine milieu, the balance of which ensures optimal fetal development, placental tolerance and pregnancy maintenance. Danger signals originating from microbial infection can trigger a maternal immune response to alter this immunological balance, thereby affecting the phenotype and function of maternal immune cells, resulting in pregnancy complications or abnormal fetal development (Fig. 5.1). Ultimately, a further understanding of these systems and their complexities may assist in optimising fetal protection in utero, thereby helping to predict and prevent subsequent neurological impairments.

Acknowledgment

The authors acknowledge support of the Eunice Kennedy Shriver National Institute of Child Health and Human Development (NICDH) P01HD054713 and 3N01 HD23342 from the Perinatal Research Branch of Eunice Kennedy Shriver NICHD, National Institutes of Health.

REFERENCES

Abrahams VM, Kim YM, Straszewski SL, Romero R, Mor G (2004) Macrophages and apoptotic cell clearance during pregnancy. *Am J Reprod Immunol* 51(4): 275–282. doi: http://dx.doi.org/10.1111/j.1600-0897.2004.00156.x.

Abrahams VM, Aldo PB, Murphy SP et al. (2008) TLR6 modulates first trimester trophoblast responses to peptidoglycan. *J Immunol* 180(9): 6035–6043. doi: http://dx.doi.org/10.4049/jimmunol.180.9.6035.

Arechavaleta-Velasco F, Gomez L, Ma Y et al. (2008) Adverse reproductive outcomes in urban women with adeno-associated virus-2 infections in early pregnancy. *Hum Reprod* 23(1): 29–36. doi: http://dx.doi.org/10.1093/humrep/dem360.

Arruvito L, Sanz M, Banham AH, Fainboim L (2007) Expansion of CD4+CD25+and FOXP3+ regulatory T cells during the follicular phase of the menstrual cycle: Implications for human reproduction. *J Immunol* 178(4): 2572–2578. doi: http://dx.doi.org/10.4049/jimmunol.178.4.2572.

Barker, D. J. (1994) Maternal and fetal origins of coronary heart disease. *J R Coll Physicians Lond* 28(6): 544–551.

Billingham RE, Brent L, Medawar, PB (1953) Actively acquired tolerance of foreign cells. *Nature* 172(4379): 603–606. doi: http://dx.doi.org/10.1038/172603a0.

Blois SM, Barrientos G, Garcia MG et al. (2008) Interaction between dendritic cells and natural killer cells during pregnancy in mice. *J Mol Med (Berl)* 86(7): 837–852. doi: http://dx.doi.org/10.1007/s00109-008-0342-2.

Brown AS, Hooton J, Schaefer CA et al. (2004) Elevated maternal interleukin-8 levels and risk of schizophrenia in adult offspring. *Am J Psychiatry* 161(5): 889–895. doi: http://dx.doi.org/10.1176/appi.ajp.161.5.889.

Brown AS, Begg MD, Gravenstein S et al. (2004) Serologic evidence of prenatal influenza in the etiology of schizophrenia. *Arch Gen Psychiatry* 61(8): 774–780. doi: http://dx.doi.org/10.1001/archpsyc.61.8.774.

Buka SL, Tsuang MT, Torrey EF, Klebanoff MA, Wagner RL, Yolken RH (2001) Maternal cytokine levels during pregnancy and adult psychosis. *Brain Behav Immun* 15(4): 411–420. doi: http://dx.doi.org/10.1006/brbi.2001.0644.

Cardenas I, Mor G, Aldo P et al. (2010) Placental viral infection sensitizes to endotoxin-induced pre-term labor: A double hit hypothesis. *Am J Reprod Immunol* 65(2): 110-117. doi: http://dx.doi.org/10.1111/j.1600-0897.2010.00908.x.

Cardenas I, Aldo P, Koga K, Means R, Lang SH, Mor G (2009) Subclinical viral infection in pregnancy lead to inflammatory process at the placenta with non-lethal fetal damage. *Am J Reprod Immunol* 61(4): 397.

Cardenas I, Means RE, Aldo P et al. (2010) Viral infection of the placenta leads to fetal inflammation and sensitization to bacterial products predisposing to preterm labor. *J Immunol* 185(2): 1248-1257. doi: http://dx.doi.org/10.4049/jimmunol.1000289.

Chaouat G, Diallo JT, Volumenie JL et al. (1997) Immune suppression and Th1/Th2 balance in pregnancy revisited: A (very) personal tribute to Tom Wegmann. *Am J Reprod Immunol* 37(6): 427–434. doi: http://dx.doi.org/10.1111/j.1600-0897.1997.tb00255.x.

Chez MG, Dowling T, Patel PB, Khanna P, Kominsky M (2007) Elevation of tumor necrosis factor-alpha in cerebrospinal fluid of autistic children. *Pediatr Neurol* 36(6): 361–365. doi: http://dx.doi.org/10.1016/j.pediatrneurol.2007.01.012.

Colbern GT, Main EK (1991) Immunology of the maternal-placental interface in normal pregnancy. *Semin Perinatol* 15(3): 196–205.

Dekel N, Gnainsky Y, Granot I, Mor G (2010) Inflammation and implantation. *Am J Reprod Immunol* 63(1): 17–21.

Espinoza J, Erez O, Romero R (2006) Preconceptional antibiotic treatment to prevent preterm birth in women with a previous preterm delivery. *Am J Obstet Gynecol* 194(3): 630–637. doi: http://dx.doi.org/10.1016/j.ajog.2005.11.050.

Gilmore JH, Jarskogm LF (1997) Exposure to infection and brain development: Cytokines in the pathogenesis of schizophrenia. *Schizophr Res* 24(3): 365–367. doi: http://dx.doi.org/10.1016/s0920-9964(96)00123-5.

Gnainsky Y, Granot I, Aldo PB et al. (2010) Local injury of the endometrium induces an inflammatory response that promotes successful implantation. *Fertil Steril* 94(6): 2030–2036. doi: http://dx.doi.org/10.1016/j.fertnstert.2010.02.022.

Hanna J, Goldman-Wohl D, Hamani Y et al. (2006) Decidual NK cells regulate key developmental processes at the human fetal-maternal interface. *Nat Med* 12(9): 1065–1074. doi: http://dx.doi.org/10.1038/nm1452.

Holmberg JC, Haddad S, Wünsche V et al. (2012). An in vitro model for the study of human implantation. *Am J Reprod Immunol* 67(2): 169–178. doi: http://dx.doi.org/10.1111/j.1600-0897.2011.01095.x.

Jasper MJ, Tremellen KP, Robertson SA (2006) Primary unexplained infertility is associated with reduced expression of the T-regulatory cell transcription factor Foxp3 in endometrial tissue. *Mol Hum Reprod* 12(5): 301–308. doi: http://dx.doi.org/10.1093/molehr/gal032.

Kim YM, Romero R, Chaiworapongsa T et al. (2004) Toll-like receptor-2 and -4 in the chorioamniotic membranes in spontaneous labor at term and in preterm parturition that are associated with chorioamnionitis. *Am J Obstet Gynecol* 191(4): 1346–1355. doi: http://dx.doi.org/10.1016/j.ajog.2004.07.009.

Koga K, Aldo PB, Mor G (2009) Toll-like receptors and pregnancy: Trophoblast as modulators of the immune response. *J Obstet Gynaecol Res* 35(2): 191–202. doi: http://dx.doi.org/10.1111/j.1447-0756.2008.00963.x.

Laskarin G, Kämmerer U, Rukavina D, Thomson AW, Fernandez N, Blois SM (2007) Antigen-presenting cells and materno-fetal tolerance: An emerging role for dendritic cells. *Am J Reprod Immunol* 58(3): 255–267. doi: http://dx.doi.org/10.1111/j.1600-0897.2007.00511.x.

Leber A, Teles A, Zenclussen AC (2010) Regulatory T cells and their role in pregnancy. *Am J Reprod Immunol* 63(6): 445–459. doi: http://dx.doi.org/10.1111/j.1600-0897.2010.00821.x.

Mackler AM, Iezza G, Akin MR, McMillan P, Yellon SM (1999) Macrophage trafficking in the uterus and cervix precedes parturition in the mouse. *Biol Reprod* 61(4): 879–883. doi: http://dx.doi.org/10.1095/biolreprod61.4.879.

Madsen-Bouterse SA, Romero R, Tarca AL et al. (2010) The transcriptome of the fetal inflammatory response syndrome. *Am J Reprod Immunol* 63(1): 73–92. doi: http://dx.doi.org/10.1111/j.1600-0897.2009.00791.x.

Manaster I, Mandelboim O (2008) The unique properties of human NK cells in the uterine mucosa. *Placenta* 29(Suppl A): S60–S66. doi: http://dx.doi.org/10.1016/j.placenta.2007.10.006.

Mantovani A, Bottazzi B, Colotta F, Sozzani S, Ruco L (1992). The origin and function of tumour associated macrophages. *Immunol Today* 13: 265–270. doi: http://dx.doi.org/10.1016/0167-5699(92)90008-U.

Mantovani A, Sica A, Locati M (2005) Macrophage polarization comes of age. *Immunity* 23(4): 344–346. doi: http://dx.doi.org/10.1016/j.immuni.2005.10.001.

Medawar PB (1948) Immunity to homologous grafted skin. III. The fate of skin homografts transplanted to the brain, to subcutaneous tissue, and to the anterior chamber of the eye. *Brit J Exp Pathol* 29: 58–69.

Meseguer M, Aplin JD, Caballero-Campo P et al. (2001) Human endometrial mucin MUC1 is up-regulated by progesterone and down-regulated in vitro by the human blastocyst. *Biol Reprod* 64(2): 590–601. doi: http://dx.doi.org/10.1095/biolreprod64.2.590.

Mills CD, Kincaid K, Alt JM, Heilman MJ, Hill AM (2000) M-1/M-2 macrophages and the Th1/Th2 paradigm. *J Immunol* 164(12): 6166–6173. doi: http://dx.doi.org/10.4049/jimmunol.164.12.6166.

Mjösberg J, Berg G, Jenmalm MC, Ernerudh J (2010) FOXP3+ regulatory T cells and T helper 1, T helper 2, and T helper 17 cells in human early pregnancy decidua. *Biol Reprod* 82(4): 698–705. doi: http://dx.doi.org/10.1095/biolreprod.109.081208.

Moffett A, Loke C (2006) Immunology of placentation in eutherian mammals. *Nat Rev Immunol* 6(8): 584–594. doi: http://dx.doi.org/10.1038/nri1897.

Mor G, Cardenas I (2010) The immune system in pregnancy: A unique complexity. *Am J Reprod Immunol* 63(6): 425–433. doi: http://dx.doi.org/10.1111/j.1600-0897.2010.00836.x.

Mor G, Romero R, Abrahams V (2006) *Macrophages and Pregnancy*. New York, Springer/ Landes BioScience.

Mor G, Cardenas I, Abrahams V, Guller S (2011) Inflammation and pregnancy: The role of the immune system at the implantation site. *Ann N Y Acad Sci* 1221: 80–87. doi: http://dx.doi.org/10.1111/j.1749-6632.2010.05938.x.

Murphy SP, Fast LD, Hanna NN, Sharma S (2005) Uterine NK cells mediate inflammation-induced fetal demise in IL-10-null mice. *J Immunol* 175(6): 4084–4090. doi: http://dx.doi.org/10.4049/jimmunol.175.6.4084.

Nagamatsu T, Schust DJ (2010) The contribution of macrophages to normal and pathological pregnancies. *Am J Reprod Immunol* 63(6): 460–471. doi: http://dx.doi.org/10.1111/j.1600-0897.2010.00813.x.

Nagamatsu T, Schust DJ (2010) The immunomodulatory roles of macrophages at the maternal-fetal interface. *Reprod Sci* 17(3): 209–218. doi: http://dx.doi.org/10.1177/1933719109349962.

Ng SC, Gilman-Sachs A, Thaker P, Beaman KD, Beer AE, Kwak-Kim J (2002) Expression of intracellular Th1 and Th2 cytokines in women with recurrent spontaneous abortion, implantation failures after IVF/ ET or normal pregnancy. *Am J Reprod Immunol* 48(2): 77–86. doi: http://dx.doi.org/10.1034/j.1600-0897.2002.01105.x.

Patterson PH (2009) Immune involvement in schizophrenia and autism: Etiology, pathology and animal models. *Behav Brain Res* 204(2): 313–321. doi: http://dx.doi.org/10.1016/j.bbr.2008.12.016.

Plaks V, Kalchenko V, Dekel N, Neeman M (2006) MRI analysis of angiogenesis during mouse embryo implantation. *Magn Reson Med* 55(5): 1013–1022. doi: http://dx.doi.org/10.1002/mrm.20881.

Plaks V, Birnberg T, Berkutzki T (2008) Uterine DCs are crucial for decidua formation during embryo implantation in mice. *J Clin Invest* 118(12): 3954–3965. doi: http://dx.doi.org/10.1172/jci36682.

Plevyak M, Hanna N, Mayer S et al. (2002) Deficiency of decidual IL-10 in first trimester missed abortion: A lack of correlation with the decidual immune cell profile. *Am J Reprod Immunol* 47(4): 242–250. doi: http://dx.doi.org/10.1034/j.1600-0897.2002.01060.x.

Racicot K, Kwon JY, Aldo P, Silasi M, Mor G (2014) Understanding the complexity of the immune system during pregnancy. *Am J Reprod Immunol* 72(2): 107–116. doi: http://dx.doi.org/10.1111/aji.12289.

Ramhorst R, Fraccaroli L, Aldo P et al. (2012) Modulation and recruitment of inducible regulatory T cells by first trimester trophoblast cells. *Am J Reprod Immunol* 67(1): 17–27. doi: http://dx.doi.org/10.1111/j.1600-0897.2011.01056.x.

Romero R, Espinoza J, Chaiworapongsa T, Kalache K (2002) Infection and prematurity and the role of preventive strategies. *Semin Neonatol* 7(4): 259–274. doi: http://dx.doi.org/10.1053/siny.2002.0121.

Saito S (2000) Cytokine network at the feto-maternal interface. *J Reprod Immunol* 47: 87–103. doi: http://dx.doi.org/10.1016/s0165-0378(00)00060-7.

Saito S, Miyazaki S, Sasaki Y (2006) *Th1/Th2 balance of the implantation site in humans.* Georgetown, Texas, Landes Bioscience/Springer Science.

Sakaguchi S, Sakaguchi N, Asano M, Itoh M, Toda M (1995) Immunologic self-tolerance maintained by activated T cells expressing IL-2 receptor alpha-chains (CD25). Breakdown of a single mechanism of self-tolerance causes various autoimmune diseases. *J Immunol* 155(3): 1151–1164.

Sakamoto Y, Moran P, Bulmer JN, Searle RF, Robson SC (2005) Macrophages and not granulocytes are involved in cervical ripening. *J Reprod Immunol* 66(2): 161–173. doi: http://dx.doi.org/10.1016/j.jri.2005.04.005.

Sasaki Y, Sakai M, Miyazaki S, Higuma S, Shiozaki A, Saito S (2004) Decidual and peripheral blood CD4+CD25+ regulatory T cells in early pregnancy subjects and spontaneous abortion cases. *Mol Hum Reprod* 10(5): 347–353. doi: http://dx.doi.org/10.1093/molehr/gah044.

Schumacher A, Wafula, PO, Bertoja AZ et al. (2007) Mechanisms of action of regulatory T cells specific for paternal antigens during pregnancy. *Obstet Gynecol* 110(5): 1137–1145. doi: http://dx.doi.org/10.1097/01.aog.0000284625.10175.31.

Shi L, Smith SEP, Malkova N, Tse D, Su Y, Patterson PH (2009) Activation of the maternal immune system alters cerebellar development in the offspring. *Brain Behav Immun* 23(1): 116–123. doi: http://dx.doi.org/10.1016/j.bbi.2008.07.012.

Simon C, Martin JC, Meseguer M, Caballero-Campo P, Valbuena D, Pellicer A (2000) Embryonic regulation of endometrial molecules in human implantation. *J Reprod Fertil* Suppl 55: 43–53.

Smith SEP, Li J, Garbett K, Mirnics K, Patterson PH (2007) Maternal immune activation alters fetal brain development through interleukin-6. *J Neurosci* 27(40): 10695–10702. doi: http://dx.doi.org/10.1523/jneurosci.2178-07.2007.

Somerset DA, Zheng Y, Kilby MD, Sansom DM, Drayson MT (2004) Normal human pregnancy is associated with an elevation in the immune suppressive CD25+ CD4+ regulatory T-cell subset. *Immunology* 112(1): 38–43. doi: http://dx.doi.org/10.1111/j.1365-2567.2004.01869.x.

Vargas DL, Nascimbene C, Krishnan C, Zimmerman AW, Pardo CA (2005) Neuroglial activation and neuroinflammation in the brain of patients with autism. *Ann Neurol* 57(1): 67–81. doi: http://dx.doi.org/10.1002/ana.20315.

Wegmann TG, Guilbert LJ (1992) Immune signaling at the maternal-fetal interface and trophoblast differentiation. *Dev Comp Immunol* 16(6): 425–430. doi: http://dx.doi.org/10.1016/0145-305x(92)90026-9.

Young A, Thomson AJ, Ledingham M, Jordan F, Greer IA, Norman JE (2002) Immunolocalization of pro-inflammatory cytokines in myometrium, cervix, and fetal membranes during human parturition at term. *Biol Reprod* 66(2): 445–449. doi: http://dx.doi.org/10.1095/biolreprod66.2.445.

Zenclussen AC, Gerlof K, Zenclussen ML (2005) Abnormal T-cell reactivity against paternal antigens in spontaneous abortion: Adoptive transfer of pregnancy-induced CD4+CD25+ T regulatory cells prevents fetal rejection in a murine abortion model. *Am J Pathol* 166(3): 811–822. doi: http://dx.doi.org/10.1016/s0002-9440(10)62302-4.

6
INFECTIONS AND THE FETAL INFLAMMATORY RESPONSE

Donald Peebles and Catherine James

Infection in pregnancy

As defined in the previous chapter, pregnancy is a time of significant immunomodulation. Traditionally considered a period of relative immunosuppression, with a shift from T helper cell 1 (Th-1) 1- to Th2-mediated immunity, pregnancy is now recognized as a complex combination of both pro- and anti-inflammatory processes. Implantation and endometrial invasion and the initiation of labor itself, are all associated with the release of pro-inflammatory cytokines and an influx of monocytes, macrophages and neutrophils to the uterus (Mor and Cardenas 2010). Conversely, established labor is associated with an immune paresis, with a reduction in major histocompatability complex class II expression and with a reduction in tumor necrosis factor alpha (TNFα) production in response to infectious challenge. This monocyte hypo-responsiveness is even more pronounced in preterm labor or preterm premature rupture of membranes (PPROM) (Lloyd et al. 2007).

Infection, classically described as invasion and multiplication of microbes accompanied by injury to host tissues, is strongly associated with preterm labor and preterm rupture of membranes (PROM). Significant evidence links the presence of pathogens in the usually sterile uterine cavity with a markedly increased risk of preterm birth. The long-term consequences of preterm birth are well documented, with 80% of children born preterm having persistent disability at 6 years of age (Marlow et al. 2005) and up to 45% showing signs of cognitive impairment by age 11 (Johnson et al. 2009). Proven bacterial infection of the amniotic fluid is predictive of poorer long-term outcomes for preterm infants; however, increasing evidence suggests that prolonged in utero exposure to inflammation is equally critical in terms of neonatal and childhood morbidity.

Inflammation, as the means by which the immune system responds to tissue damage, can be both infective and sterile. It can also be physiological, for example, ovarian follicle rupture, menstruation and implantation (Gotsch et al. 2007). Inflammation of the amnion and chorion, chorioamnionitis, is defined by the presence of an inflammatory infiltrate on histological examination (Fig. 6.1). Similarly, funisitis is the result of a migratory infiltrate of polymorphs from the lumen of the umbilical vessels into the vessel walls (Pacora et al. 2002, Fig. 6.2). Chorioamnionitis is frequently subclinical during pregnancy, both when associated with preterm labor and when present at term. However, there is often a marked inflammatory syndrome evident in both the fetus and the neonate, the presence of which seems to herald

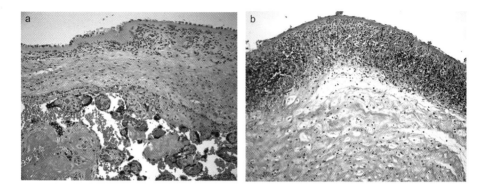

Fig. 6.1. Histological sections of fetal membranes showing inflammatory infiltrate (blue poly-morphonuclear leukocytes) characteristic of severe chorioamnionitis. (a) Neutrophils migrating toward the amniotic cavity. (b) Necrotizing chorioamnionitis characterized by severe acute inflammation and focal necrosis. Reproduced from *Surg Pathol Clin: Placental Pathol* 6 (1): 33–60, with permission from WB Saunders. A colour version of this figure can be seen in the plate section at the end of the book.

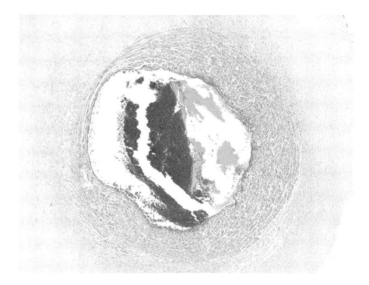

Fig. 6.2. Histological section of umbilical cord showing inflammatory infiltrate characteristic of funisitis. In this severe fetal inflammatory response, fetal neutrophils infiltrate the umbilical vascula-ture and expand into the Wharton substance. Later stages (necrotizing funisitis) are defined by con-centric bands around the vessels.

significant neonatal morbidity. It is therefore perhaps somewhat counterintuitive that preterm fetuses, with histological evidence of chorioamnionitis, are more likely to survive the neonatal period than those born preterm without evidence of chorioamnionitis (Gotsch et al. 2007). This suggests that inflammation, while associated with end organ damage in the fetal inflam-matory syndrome, also has a restorative role in preterm neonates.

Intrauterine infection

There is increasing clinical and experimental evidence that the uterine cavity is sterile in pregnancy and that bacterial presence in the intrauterine cavity is associated with both PPROM and spontaneous preterm labor with intact membranes. Animal models with sheep (Bieghs et al. 2010), mice (Agrawal and Hirsch 2012), rabbits (Gotsch et al. 2007) and monkeys (Waldorf et al. 2011) demonstrate that intrauterine inoculation with either live bacteria or toxins can initiate preterm labor.

Microbiological examination of amniotic fluid has been used to show an association between the presence of bacteria and subsequent risk of preterm labor (Agrawal and Hirsch 2012). Detection of bacteria and indeed viruses, in amniotic fluid and fetal membranes has traditionally been problematic. The vast majority of bacteria associated with preterm birth are obligate anaerobes, difficult to culture with conventional techniques. When amniotic fluid is examined using molecular microbiological techniques, based on broad range 16s polymerase chain reaction (PCR), bacteria have been detected in 50% of samples from women with PPROM. These findings are shown to be predictive of lower birthweights and increased risk of both respiratory distress syndrome and necrotizing enterocolitis in the neonate (DiGiulio et al. 2010).

Conventional culture of fetal membranes is also poorly correlative with histological chorioamnionitis. Again, in these circumstances 16s PCR has been used to increase sensitivity when investigating the presence of bacteria. Furthermore, the addition of species-specific PCR assays increases the sensitivity still further (Jones et al. 2009). Examination of placental, cord and membrane tissue with 16s and species-specific PCR after vaginal delivery at term often reveals the presence of bacteria, most commonly *ureaplasma parvum* and *lactobacillus*; however, bacteria are absent at pre-labor Cesarean section at term. This suggests that labor itself is associated with ascending migration of bacteria into the uterine cavity.

After PPROM, or spontaneous preterm labor, there is greater variety in the species of bacteria detected by molecular microbiology techniques and the proportion of patients with multiple species present is far higher. This is directly correlative with the presence of chorioamnionitis (Jones et al. 2009). Moreover, recent data have shown that the membranes and trophoblast express a range of pattern recognition molecules, suggesting that a direct inflammatory response, by these tissues, is likely (Choi et al. 2012).

Antibiotics to prevent preterm birth and treat threatened preterm labor

The use of antibiotics either prophylactically to prevent preterm birth or to treat clinically suspected ascending infection is the subject of intense debate. Given the strong association between clinical infection and preterm birth, it is not surprising that the use of antibiotics in this context has attracted significant research attention.

Studies focusing on empirical antibiotic use and targeted therapies have produced mixed results (Subramaniam et al. 2012). Hauth et al. showed that treating women at a high risk of delivering preterm with metronidazole and erythromycin for bacterial vaginosis before 24 weeks' gestation reduces the risk of a subsequent preterm birth (Hauth et al. 1995). In contrast, women enrolled in the PREMET trial, who were treated with metronidazole after a positive fetal fibronectin test, were more likely to deliver preterm than those treated with placebo (Shennan et al. 2006) and the Medical Research Council ORACLE II study revealed a higher incidence of cerebral palsy at 7 years of age in children of women who received erythromycin for PPROM (Kenyon et al. 2008).

The heterogeneous methodologies used in these previous studies may be one reason for the varied evidence regarding antibiotic use to treat and prevent preterm birth (Lamont et al. 2011). It is also notable that, to date, only the ORACLE studies (I and II) include data regarding the long-term outcome of children exposed to antibiotics in this context; it is at least in part this shortfall that ensures antibiotic use in these women remains controversial.

Viral infections and inflammation

Maternal systemic viral infection is widely accepted to be a cause of fetal and neonatal morbidity; for example, maternal varicella zoster infection is associated with the fetal varicella syndrome (Mandelbrot 2012) and maternal cytomegalovirus (CMV) is associated with congenital neurological deficit (Visentin et al. 2012).

Human immunodeficiency virus (HIV) infection is widely reported as an independent risk factor for preterm delivery. However, a recent report suggests that this relationship may not be as straightforward as previously envisaged; as in a large cohort study, Ndirangu et al. found an association between maternal HIV infection and low birthweight, especially in the presence of severe immunosuppression, but not with preterm delivery (Ndirangu et al. 2012). The authors suggest that the reliability of gestational age data in previous studies and more detailed attention to possible confounding factors may account for these contradictory findings.

Both clinical and experimental evidence suggest that viruses are capable of engaging a fetal immune response. Primary CMV infection in pregnancy is associated with the presence of CMV DNA in the amniotic fluid. Furthermore, where CMV DNA is present, it is associated with increased concentrations of the pro-inflammatory cytokines TNFα, IL-1β, IL-12 and IL-17 and chemokines CCL2, CCL4 and CXCL10 (Scott et al. 2012). Raised IL-1β, together with raised IL-13 and increased levels of chemokine MCP-1 and colony stimulating factor vasculature endothelial growth factor (VEGF) has also been shown in the developing CNS of mouse pups following maternal trans-peritoneal inoculation with the synthetic viral double-stranded RNA analogue poly(I:C) (polyriboinosinic-polyribocytidylic acid) (Arrode-Brusés and Brusés 2012). In contrast, Gervasi et al. found no difference in the concentration of IL-6 in amniotic fluid where viral DNA was detected (Human Herpes Virus 6 [HHV6], CMV, Parvovirus B 19 [PB19] and Epstein Barr Virus [EBV]), although they did report an increase in the chemokine CXCL-10 (Gervasi et al. 2012). The authors acknowledge that IL-6, a cytokine associated with bacterial infection, may not be an appropriate marker of viral infection. To date, co-infection of the intrauterine cavity with both bacteria and viruses has not been fully explored in the literature.

Peripheral infection and inflammation

Periodontal disease is strongly associated with preterm birth (Khader and Ta'ani 2005, Offenbacher et al. 2006, Offenbacher et al. 2009). However, the mechanism remains elusive. Moreover, treating periodontal disease does not reduce the risk of spontaneous preterm birth

(Michalowicz and Hodges 2006, Macones et al. 2010, Polyzos et al. 2010). There are two main hypotheses to explain the connection between periodontal disease and preterm birth that (1) local host defense systems in the periodontium release cytokines into the systemic circulation, which irritate the uterus resulting in contractions; and (2) the pathogens causing the periodontitis disseminate hematogenously and directly initiate an immune response in the genital tract (Goepfert et al. 2004).

As Goepfert et al. showed that periodontitis is not independently associated with clinical chorioamnionitis, microbial growth on cord blood or placental cultures and raised IL-6 in cord plasma (Goepfert et al. 2004), this evidence does not support the hematogenous dissemination of pathogens hypothesis. However, it is notable that Goepfert et al. used conventional microbial culture techniques rather than molecular techniques. It would therefore be illuminating to see what, if any, correlation there is with placental and cord blood bacterial prevalence and diversity when these samples are examined using contemporary molecular microbiology techniques.

Evidence for a fetal immune system response

It is clear that the fetus can orchestrate its own immune response. Fetuses exposed to PPROM and ascending infection show increased neutrophil and monocyte activation and high circulating concentrations of IL-6, IFNγ and CRP. These pro-inflammatory cytokines do not cross the placenta, so are almost certainly of fetal/placental origin (Aaltonen et al. 2005). Furthermore, functional regulatory cells are detectable in the thymus at between 14 and 17 weeks' gestation (Gotsch et al. 2007). Th1 cells are detected in cord blood and they increase in response to infection. This response correlates well with clinical evidence of maternal infection and has also been shown to be proportional in relation to the rupture of membranes in PPROM (Gotsch et al. 2007).

Classically, IL-6 is secreted by macrophages in response to pathogen engagement with pattern recognition receptors, including Toll-like receptors (TLRs). The role of these receptors themselves in preterm labor is under consideration. TLR2, a ligand for gram-positive bacteria, is up-regulated in both chorioamnionitis and preterm labor. Conversely, antagonists of the TLR4 receptor (a gram-negative ligand) significantly reduce the risk of inflammation and preterm labor in both mice and monkey models (Agrawal and Hirsch 2012). IL-6 secretion induces acute phase proteins and also plays a critical role in the regulation of hematopoiesis by promoting the survival of hematopoietic stem cells and their progenitors. In addition, IL-6 regulates the differentiation and proliferation of hematopoietic cells at a variety of lineages and maturation, including stimulating the proliferation of macrophages. These effects are achieved in synergy with IL-3 (Rodríguez, Bernad & Aracil 2004).

Romero et al. have shown that fetuses with a plasma IL-6 concentration greater than 11 pg/ml have a higher median corrected white blood cell count and a higher corrected neutrophil count and are more likely to have a frank neutrophilia (Romero et al. 2011). This distinct hematological profile is an example of a systemic response in the fetus to the presence of pathogens. In addition to these regulatory effects, elevated fetal plasma IL-6 is associated with imminent preterm labor, suggesting that the fetal immune response is directly involved in the initiation of labor (Romero and Chaiworapongsa 2003).

The fetal inflammatory response syndrome

Fetal inflammatory response syndrome (FIRS) is a multi-system inflammatory syndrome that develops in response to stimuli encountered during fetal life. Neonates born with FIRS have a distinct clinical phenotype; they are more likely to require extended neonatal unit admissions and experience significant perinatal morbidity. In addition, the risk of perinatal mortality is higher in these infants. These effects are independent of gestational age at birth.

FIRS can be triggered by any significant immune trigger to the fetus; the most common association is with preterm labor and PPROM, but viral infection of the intrauterine cavity, for example, with CMV, can also be causative (Gotsch et al. 2007). Non-infective events may also trigger FIRS; for example, rhesus alloimmunization (Vaisbuch et al. 2011). The severity of FIRS seems to correlate with the presence of bacteria in the amniotic fluid, with a milder syndrome being observed in fetuses without intra-amniotic infection and a more severe syndrome affecting those with proven intra-amniotic infection (Lee et al. 2007).

Gotsch et al. suggest that FIRS is a direct fetal counterpart of the systemic immune response syndrome (SIRS) seen in adults. It is the most common cause of mortality in adult patients admitted to the intensive therapy unit with sepsis. SIRS is defined by clinical parameters, (e.g. blood pressure), that are not easily applicable to the fetus (Gotsch et al. 2007). Consequently, diagnosis of FIRS is defined by the presence of an IL-6 concentration above or equal to 11 ng/l in the fetal plasma.

Fetal inflammatory response syndrome and lung disease

FIRS itself is associated with an increased risk of chronic lung disease (CLD) and this risk is higher still in fetuses with FIRS superimposed on histological chorioamnionitis or funisitis. Nevertheless, this association is somewhat controversial, with questions raised about variations in methodology, for example, adjustments for birthweight and definitions of CLD and chorioamnionitis used (Dessardo et al. 2012). These concerns notwithstanding, it seems likely that the presence of chorioamnionitis results in a more extreme lung injury than accounted for by preterm birth alone (Jobe and Ikegami 2001).

Despite the apparent association with CLD, it is suggested that chorioamnionitis and FIRS may be in some way *protective* of the lungs of preterm infants. Chorioamnionitis promotes lung maturity in fetal lambs (Kallapur et al. 2001) and funisitis reduces the risk of respiratory distress syndrome (RDS) in infants born before 32 weeks' gestation (Lee et al. 2011). This may be related to the direct increase in surfactant proteins and increased compliance observed after intra-amniotic inoculation with lipopolysaccharide (LPS). This increase in surfactant proteins is mediated by prostaglandins (Westover et al. 2012). Furthermore, it has been suggested that surfactant protein A itself may be able to modulate intrauterine inflammatory mediators (Salminen et al. 2011), adding to the evidence that the fetal immune response is directly involved with the initiation of preterm labor.

Although FIRS may reduce the risk of RDS in preterm infants, it is associated with an increased risk of bronchopulmonary dysplasia (BPD). Indeed, increased cord plasma concentration of IL-6 is an independent risk factor for BPD and suggests that the pathogenesis of BPD is likely to be initiated before birth in infants with funisitis and BPD (Yoon et al. 1999) either by exposure to pro-inflammatory cytokines in the amniotic fluid or by the systemic immune response of the fetus itself (Jobe and Ikegami 2001). High concentrations of pro-inflammtory IL-1β are found in aspirates of tracheal fluid on the first day of intubation in fetuses with chorioamnionitis. These infants are more likely to develop BPD (Gotsch et al. 2007), an observation which supports the hypothesis that the pathogenesis of BPD can be traced back to exposure to pro-inflammatory cytokines in utero.

FETAL INFLAMMATORY RESPONSE SYNDROME AND THE BRAIN

FIRS has been described as a firm link between antenatal infection, white matter damage and persistent motor abnormalities (Dammann and Kuban 2002). There is a strong correlation between high IL-6 concentrations in umbilical cord plasma and white matter damage in the fetal brain. Periventricular leukomalacia (PVL) (Fig. 6.3) is associated with sepsis, intraventricular hemorrhage and perinatal death (Mittendorf et al. 2003). For neonates with histological chorioamnionitis, born within an hour of membrane rupture, the presence of funisitis has been shown to cause an 11-fold increase in the risk of ultrasound-defined white matter damage. (Dammann and Kuban 2002). Furthermore, both histological and clinical chorioamnionitis are associated with cerebral palsy (CP), regardless of gestational age (Gotsch et al. 2007).

In seeking to disentangle the contributions of pre- and postnatal systemic inflammation to the risk of CP and severe early cognitive development, the extremely low gestational age newborns (ELGAN) study has made considerable inroads. This prospective study of over 1500 infants, born before 28 weeks' gestation between 2002 and 2004, has provided direct supporting evidence that microorganisms can increase the risk of white matter damage

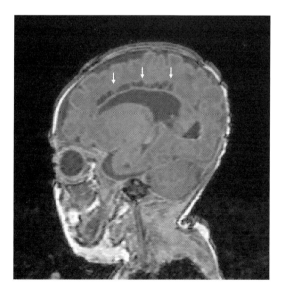

Fig. 6.3. Magnetic resonance image (sagittal plane, T1 weighted spin echo sequence) of a neonatal brain showing cystic periventricular leukomalacia (PVL)—necrotic regions (white arrows) near to the lateral ventricles.

(WMD) in extremely preterm infants. In their microbiological and histological examinations of collected placentas, not only did they confirm that inflammation of the chorionic plate and chorion/decidua were linked with the risk of diffuse WMD and diparetic CP, the recovery of low-virulence micro-organisms (some typical of skin microflora) from the placenta was predictive of both quadriparetic and diparetic CP, particularly when aligned with placenta inflammation (Leviton et al. 2010).

Of all neonatal conditions linked to poor neurological outcome in preterm infants, PVL has the strongest association. Neonates with PVL are more likely to develop a variety of neurological complications, ranging from neuromotor disorders to cognitive limitations and behavioral difficulties. Furthermore, fetuses exposed to infection, but who do not go on to develop PVL, may experience neurological damage related to preterm birth; this may include neuronal damage or apoptosis and abnormalities in synaptogenesis and neurotransmitters (Dammann and Kuban 2002).

Cerebral palsy, which often manifests after PVL, is associated with several immune-related polymorphisms in preterm neonates: endothelial NO synthetase, factor VIII, plasminigen activation factor and lymphoprotein A (Gotsch et al. 2007). Additionally, CP is correlative with increased concentrations of IL-6 and IL-8 in amniotic fluid and increased concentrations of TNFα and matrix metalloproteinase 8 (MMP-8) in either amniotic fluid or cord blood (Gotsch et al. 2007). As discussed in Chapter 11, the administration of magnesium sulfate to women at very high risk of preterm delivery has been shown to confer a neuroprotective effect (Doyle et al. 2009) and may reduce the risk of CP (Kenyon and Peebles 2011). However, as yet no single optimal regime has been described (Doyle et al. 2009).

While exposure to amniotic infection and high concentrations of pro-inflammatory cytokines in amniotic fluid is associated with fetal and early neonatal cerebral tissue injury, the role of cytokines in postnatal tissue damage is unclear (Dessardo et al. 2012). It seems likely that the pathophysiology of CP may vary with gestational age at birth (Gotsch et al. 2007). Nevertheless, integrating postnatal cytokine data does not seem to improve the predictive values of models constructed using clinical variables. This implies that in contrast to the pathogenesis of PVL developed in the antenatal period, changes in cytokine concentrations may be in response to clinical variables, rather than the other way around (Dessardo et al. 2012).

FETAL INFLAMMATORY RESPONSE SYNDROME IN OTHER ORGAN SYSTEMS

The significant effects of FIRS on the brain and lungs, as considered above, have been well characterized. Increasingly, however, FIRS is becoming recognized as a truly multisystemic syndrome. As evidenced, retinopathy of prematurity is more severe in neonates affected by FIRS and neonatal transient hypothyroxinaemia is associated with histological evidence of chorioamnionitis (Gantert et al. 2010). An association between chorioamnionitis and hepatitis and abnormal lipid profiles has also been described in sheep (Bieghs et al. 2010). Fetal sheep have been shown to develop dermatitis in response to intra-amniotic infection (Kemp et al. 2011). FIRS dermatitis has been described as the fetal counterpart of chorioamnionitis (Kim et al. 2006) and fetuses with chorioamnionitis have increased expression of TLR2 and TLR4 in both the epidermis and the dermal/epidermal junction (Gotsch et al. 2007).

The influence of FIRS on the fetal cardiovascular system has been proposed as a causative mechanism for PVL. Neonates with histological chorioamnionitis have a lower mean and diastolic blood pressure and mean blood pressure is inversely proportional to cord plasma IL-6 concentrations. It has been suggested that this combination of parameters is likely to have developed in utero. Increased left ventricular compliance is well recognized in SIRS and has also been described in FIRS (Romero et al. 2004, Di Naro et al. 2010). This is a compensatory mechanism and if the fetus is unable to modify ventricular compliance, cardiac output may not be maintained. This would result in a combination of hypotension and cerebral ischemia in utero and together with local inflammation in the brain, may exacerbate brain injury (Gotsch et al. 2007, Di Naro et al. 2010).

Oligohydramnios is also common in infants with PPROM and chorioamnionitis (Yoon, et al. 1999), with an amniotic fluid index of five or below associated with a higher probability of histological or clinical chorioamnionitis, higher concentrations of cord plasma and amniotic fluid IL-6 and higher IL-1β and TNFα in the amniotic fluid. Combined, these features have been presented as evidence for fetal renal tract involvement in FIRS (Gotsch et al. 2007). Recently, Galinsky et al. have shown that intra-amniotic injection of LPS is associated with a reduction in the number of nephrons in fetal sheep. Interestingly, there was no difference in the degree of renal inflammation between those fetuses exposed to LPS and their controls (Galinsky et al. 2011). Although no difference in *inflammation* was demonstrated, these data do show that the fetal renal tract makes a significant response to infective stimuli.

Conclusion

Substantial clinical and experimental evidence has shown that the fetal immune system may be engaged during pregnancy, both directly in response to pathogenic stimuli and indirectly as a result of a maternal inflammatory response. Inflammation in fetal life has significant implications for both the immediate neonatal period and the long-term well-being of the child. Despite the widely described consequences of chorioamnionitis and FIRS, the optimal time for delivery of affected fetuses has yet to be determined. Progesterone and cervical cerclage are both used to delay the onset of labor, however, the implications of delayed delivery in the presence of infection are unknown and the risks of continued exposure to inflammatory stimuli must be weighed against the risks of preterm birth.

REFERENCES

Aaltonen R, Heikkinen T, Hakala K, Laine K, Alanen A (2005) Transfer of proinflammatory cytokines across term placenta. *Obset Gynecol* 106: 802–807. doi: http://dx.doi.org/10.1097/01.aog.0000178750. 84837.ed.

Agrawal V, Hirsch E (2012) Intrauterine infection and preterm labor. *Semin Fetal Neonatal Med* 17(1): 12–19. doi: http://dx.doi.org/10.1016/j.siny.2011.09.001.

Arrode-Brusés G, Brusés JL (2012) Maternal immune activation by poly(I:C) induces expression of cytokines IL-1beta and IL-13, chemokine MCP-1 and colony stimulating factor VEGF in fetal mouse brain. *J Neuroinflammation* 9(1): 83. doi: http://dx.doi.org/10.1186/1742-2094-9-83.

Bieghs V, Vlassaks E, Custers A et al. (2010) Chorioamnionitis induced hepatic inflammation and disturbed lipid metabolism in fetal sheep. *Pediatr Res* 68(6): 466–472. doi: http://dx.doi.org/10.1203/ pdr.0b013e3181f70eeb.

Choi SJ, Jung SH, Eom M, Han KH, Chung IB, Kim SK (2012) Immunohistochemical distribution of toll-like receptor 4 in preterm fetal membrane. *J Obstet Gynaecol Res* 38(1): 108–112. doi: http://dx.doi.org/10.1111/j.1447-0756.2011.01626.x.

Dammann O, Kuban K (2002) Perinatal infection, fetal inflammatory response, white matter damage, and cognitive limitations in children born preterm. *Ment Retard Dev D R* 8: 46–50. doi: http://dx.doi.org/10.1002/mrdd.10005.

Dessardo NS, Mustać E, Dessardo S et al. (2012) Chorioamnionitis and chronic lung disease of prematurity: A path analysis of causality. *Am J Perinatol* 29(2): 133–140. doi: http://dx.doi.org/10.1055/s-0031-1295654.

Di Naro E, Cromi A, Ghezzi F, Giocolano A, Caringella A, Loverro G. (2010) Myocardial dysfunction in fetuses exposed to intraamniotic infection: New insights from tissue Doppler and strain imaging. *Am J Obstet Gynecol* 203: 459.e1–459.e7. doi: http://dx.doi.org/10.1016/j.ajog.2010.06.033.

DiGiulio DB, Romero R, Kusanovic JP et al. (2010) Prevalence and diversity of microbes in the amniotic fluid, the fetal inflammatory response, and pregnancy outcome in women with preterm pre-labor rupture of membranes. *Am J Reprod Immunol* 64(1): 38–57. doi: http://dx.doi.org/10.1111/j.1600-0897.2010.00830.x.

Doyle LW, Crowther CA, Middleton P, Marret S, Rouse D (2009) Magnesium sulphate for women at risk of preterm birth for neuroprotection of the fetus. *Cochrane Database of Systematic Reviews* (Online) 1: CD004661.

Galinsky R, Moss TJM, Gubhaju L, Hooper SB, Black MJ, & Polglase GR (2011) Effect of intra-amniotic lipopolysaccharide on nephron number in preterm fetal sheep. *Am J Physiol Renal Physiol* 301(2): F280–F285. doi: http://dx.doi.org/10.1152/ajprenal.00066.2011.

Gantert M, Been JV, Gavilanes AWD, Garnier Y, Zimmermann LJI, Kramer BW (2010) Chorioamnionitis: A multiorgan disease of the fetus? *J Perinatol* 30: S21–S30. doi: http://dx.doi.org/10.1038/jp.2010.96.

Gervasi M-T, Romero R, Bracalente G et al. (2012) Viral invasion of the amniotic cavity (VIAC) in the midtrimester of pregnancy. *J Matern Fetal Neonatal Med* [Epub ahead of print]. doi: http://dx.doi.org/10.3109/14767058.2012.683899.

Goepfert AR, Jeffcoat MK, Andrews WW et al. (2004) Periodontal disease and upper genital tract inflammation in early spontaneous preterm birth. *Obstet Gynecol* 104(4): 777–783. doi: http://dx.doi.org/10.1097/01.aog.0000139836.47777.6d.

Gotsch F, Romero R, Kusanovic JP et al. (2007) The fetal inflammatory response syndrome. *Clin Obstet Gynecol* 50(3): 652–683. doi: http://dx.doi.org/10.1097/grf.0b013e31811ebef6.

Gündoğan F, De Paepe ME (2013) Ascending infection: Acute chorioamnionitis. Surgical pathology clinics. *Placental Pathology* 6(1): 33–60. doi: http://dx.doi.org/10.1016/j.path.2012.11.002.

Hauth JC, Goldenberg RL, Andrews WW, DuBard MB, Copper RL (1995) Reduced incidence of preterm delivery with metronidazole and erythromycin in women with bacterial vaginosis. *N Engl J Med* 333(26): 1732–1736. doi: http://dx.doi.org/10.1056/nejm199512283332603.

Jobe A, Ikegami M (2001) Antenatal infection/inflammation and postnatal lung maturation and injury. *Respir Res* 2: 27–32. doi: http://dx.doi.org/10.1186/rr35.

Johnson S, Hennessy EM, Smith R, Trikic R, Wolke D, Marlow, N (2009) Academic attainment and special educational needs in extremely preterm children at 11 years of age: The EPICure study. *Arch Dis Child* 94(4): F283–F289. doi: http://dx.doi.org/10.1136/adc.2008.152793.

Jones HE, Harris KA, Azizia M et al. (2009) Differing prevalence and diversity of bacterial species in fetal membranes from very preterm and term labor. *PLoS ONE* 4(12): e8205. doi: http://dx.doi.org/10.1371/journal.pone.0008205.

Kallapur S, Willet K, Jobe A (2001) Intra-amniotic endotoxin: Chorioamnionitis precedes lung maturation in preterm lambs. *Am J Physiol Lung Cell Mol Physiol* 280: L527–L536.

Kemp MW, Saito M, Kallapur SG et al. (2011) Inflammation of the fetal ovine skin following in utero exposure to Ureaplasma parvum. *Reprod Sci* 18(11): 1128–1137. doi: http://dx.doi.org/10.1177/1933719111408114.

Kenyon, AP, Peebles D (2011) Myth: Tocolysis for prevention of preterm birth has a major role in modern obstetrics. *Semin Fetal Neonatal Med* 16(5): 242–246. doi: http://dx.doi.org/10.1016/j.siny.2011.04.008.

Kenyon S, Pike K, Jones DR et al. (2008) Childhood outcomes after prescription of antibiotics to pregnant women with spontaneous preterm labour: 7-year follow-up of the ORACLE II trial. *Lancet* 372: 1319–1327. doi: http://dx.doi.org/10.1016/s0140-6736(08)61203-9.

Khader DYS, Ta'ani Q (2005) Periodontal diseases and the risk of preterm birth and low birthweight: A meta-analysis. *J Peridontol* 76(2): 161–165. doi: http://dx.doi.org/10.1902/jop.2005.76.2.161.

Kim YM, Romero R, Chaiworapongsa T, Espinoza J, Mor G, Kim CJ (2006) Dermatitis as a component of the fetal inflammatory response syndrome is associated with activation of Toll-like receptors in epidermal keratinocytes. *Histopathology* 49(5) 506–514. doi: http://dx.doi.org/10.1111/j.1365-2559. 2006.02542.x.

Lamont RF, Nhan-Chang C-L, Sobel JD, Workowski K, Conde-Agudelo A, Romero R (2011) Treatment of abnormal vaginal flora in early pregnancy with clindamycin for the prevention of spontaneous preterm birth: A systematic review and meta-analysis. *Am J Obstet Gynecol* 205(3): 177–190. doi: http://dx.doi. org/10.1016/j.ajog.2011.03.047.

Lee J, Oh KJ, Park C-W, Park JS, Jun JK, Yoon BH (2011) The presence of funisitis is associated with a decreased risk for the development of neonatal respiratory distress syndrome. *Placenta* 32(3): 235–240. doi: http://dx.doi.org/10.1016/j.placenta.2010.11.006.

Lee S, Romero R, Jung H, Park C, Park JS, Yoon BH (2007) The intensity of the fetal inflammatory response in intraamniotic inflammation with and without microbial invasion of the amniotic cavity. *Am J Obstet Gynecol* 197: 294.e1–294.e6. doi: http://dx.doi.org/10.1016/j.ajog.2007.07.006.

Leviton A, Allred EN, Kuban KC et al. (2010) Microbiologic and histologic characteristics of the extremely preterm infant's placenta predict white matter damage and later cerebral palsy. The ELGAN study. *Pediatr Res* 67(1): 95–101. doi: http://dx.doi.org/10.1203/PDR.0b013e3181bf5fab.

Lloyd J, Allen M, Azizia M, Klein N, Peebles D (2007) Monocyte major histocompatibility complex class II expression in term and preterm labor. *Obstet Gynecol* 110(6): 1335–1342. doi: http://dx.doi. org/10.1097/01.aog.0000289226.08442.e1.

Macones GA, Parry S, Nelson DB et al. (2010) Treatment of localized periodontal disease in pregnancy does not reduce the occurrence of preterm birth: Results from the Periodontal Infections and Prematurity Study (PIPS). *Am J Obstet Gynecol* 202(2): 147.e1–147.e8. doi: http://dx.doi.org/10.1016/j.ajog.2009.10.892.

Mandelbrot L (2012) Fetal varicella–diagnosis, management, and outcome. *Prenat Diagn* 32(6): 511–518. doi: http://dx.doi.org/10.1002/pd.3843.

Marlow N, Hennessy EM, Bracewell MA, Wolke D (2007) Motor and executive function at 6 years of age after extremely preterm birth. *Pediatrics* 120(4): 793–804. doi: http://dx.doi.org/10.1542/peds.2007-0440.

Michalowicz B, Hodges J (2006) Treatment of periodontal disease and the risk of preterm birth. *N Engl J Med* 355: 1885–1894. doi: http://dx.doi.org/10.1056/nejmoa062249.

Mittendorf R, Montag A, MacMillan W et al. (2003) Components of the systemic fetal inflammatory response syndrome as predictors of impaired neurologic outcomes in children. *Am J Obstet Gynecol* 188: 1438–1446. doi: http://dx.doi.org/10.1067/mob.2003.380.

Mor G, & Cardenas I (2010) The immune system in pregnancy: A unique complexity. *Am J Reprod Immunol* 63(6): 425–433. doi: http://dx.doi.org/10.1111/j.1600-0897.2010.00836.x.

Ndirangu J, Newell M-L, Bland RM, Thorne C (2012) Maternal HIV infection associated with small-for-gestational age infants but not preterm births: Evidence from rural South Africa. *Hum Reprod* 27(6): 1846–1856. doi: http://dx.doi.org/10.1093/humrep/des090.

Offenbacher S, Beck JD, Jared HL et al. & the Maternal Oral Therapy to Reduce Obstetric Risk (MOTOR) Investigators. (2009) Effects of periodontal therapy on rate of preterm delivery: A randomized controlled trial. *Obstet Gynecol* 114(3): 551–559. doi: http://dx.doi.org/10.1097/aog.0b013e3181b1341f.

Offenbacher S, Boggess KA, Murtha AP et al. (2006) Progressive periodontal disease and risk of very preterm delivery. *Obstet Gynecol* 107(1): 29–36. doi: http://dx.doi.org/10.1097/01.aog.0000190212.87012.96.

Pacora P, Chaiworapongsa T, Maymon E et al. (2002) Funisitis and chorionic vasculitis: The histological counterpart of the fetal inflammatory response syndrome. *J Matern-Feto Neo Med* 11: 18–25. doi: http:// dx.doi.org/10.1080/713605445.

Polyzos NP, Polyzos IP, Zavos A et al. (2010) Obstetric outcomes after treatment of periodontal disease during pregnancy: Systematic review and meta-analysis. *BMJ* 341: c7017. doi: http://dx.doi.org/10.1136/ bmj.c7017.

Rodríguez MDC, Bernad A, Aracil M (2004) Interleukin-6 deficiency affects bone marrow stromal precursors, resulting in defective hematopoietic support. *Blood* 103(9): 3349–3354. doi: http://dx.doi. org/10.1182/blood-2003-10-3438.

Romero R, & Chaiworapongsa T (2003) Micronutrients and intrauterine infection, preterm birth and the fetal inflammatory response syndrome. *J Nutr* 133(5 Suppl 2): 1668S–1673S.

Romero R, Espinoza J, Gonçalves L et al. (2004) Fetal cardiac dysfunction in preterm premature rupture of membranes. *J Matern Fetal Neonatal Med* 16(3): 146–157. doi: http://dx.doi.org/10.1080/jmf.16.3.146.157.

Romero R, Savasan ZA, Chaiworapongsa T et al. (2011) Hematologic profile of the fetus with systemic inflammatory response syndrome. *J Perinat Med* 40(1): 19–32. doi: http://dx.doi.org/10.1515/ jpm.2011.100.

Salminen A, Vuolteenaho R, Paananen R, Ojaniemi M, Hallman M (2011) Surfactant protein A modulates the lipopolysaccharide-induced inflammatory response related to preterm birth. *Cytokine* 56(2): 442–449. doi: http://dx.doi.org/10.1016/j.cyto.2011.07.025.

Scott GM, Chow SSW, Craig ME et al. (2012) Cytomegalovirus infection during pregnancy with maternofetal transmission induces a proinflammatory cytokine bias in placenta and amniotic fluid. *J Infect Dis* 205(8): 1305–1310. doi: http://dx.doi.org/10.1093/infdis/jis186.

Shennan A, Crawshaw S, Briley A et al. (2006) A randomised controlled trial of metronidazole for the prevention of preterm birth in women positive for cervicovaginal fetal fibronectin: The PREMET Study. *BJOG-Int J Obstet Gy* 113(1): 65–74. doi: http://dx.doi.org/10.1111/j.1471-0528.2005.00788.x.

Subramaniam A, Abramovici A, Andrews WW, Tita AT (2012) Antimicrobials for preterm birth prevention: An overview. *Infect Dis Obstet Gynecol* 2012: 157159. doi: http://dx.doi.org/10.1155/2012/157159.

Vaisbuch E, Romero R, Gomez R et al. (2011) An elevated fetal interleukin-6 concentration can be observed in fetuses with anemia due to Rh alloimmunization: Implications for the understanding of the fetal inflammatory response syndrome. *J Matern Fetal Neonatal Med* 24(3): 391–396. doi: http://dx.doi.org/10.3109/14767058.2010.507294.

Visentin S, Manara R, Milanese L et al. (2012) Early primary CMV infection in pregnancy: Maternal hyperimmuneglobulin therapy improves children's outcome at one year. *Clin Infect Dis* Advance. Access Online 10.1093/cid/cis423.

Waldorf KMA, Gravett MG, McAdams RM et al. (2011) Choriodecidual group B streptococcal inoculation induces fetal lung injury without intra-amniotic infection and preterm labor in Macaca nemestrina. *PLoS ONE* 6(12): e28972. doi: http://dx.doi.org/10.1371/journal.pone.0028972.

Westover AJ, Hooper SB, Wallace MJ, Moss TJM (2012) Prostaglandins mediate the fetal pulmonary response to intrauterine inflammation. *Am J Physiol Lung Cell Mol Physiol* 302(7): L664–L678. doi: http://dx.doi.org/10.1152/ajplung.00297.2011.

Yoon B, Kim Y, Romero R et al. (1999) Association of oligohydramnios in women with preterm premature rupture of membranes with an inflammatory response in fetal, amniotic, and maternal compartments. *Am J Obstet Gynecol* 181(4): 784–788. doi: http://dx.doi.org/10.1016/s0002-9378(99)70301-7.

Yoon B, Romero R, Kim K, Park J (1999) A systemic fetal inflammatory response and the development of bronchopulmonary dysplasia. *Am J Obstet Gynecol* 181(4): 773–779. doi: http://dx.doi.org/10.1016/s0002-9378(99)70299-1.

7
CEREBRAL ISCHAEMIA AND WHITE MATTER INJURY

Suresh Victor and Michael Weindling

Cerebral white matter injury in the preterm infant is of enormous public health importance. Nearly 9000 infants are born every year with birthweight below 1500g in England and Wales alone (Office of National Statistics, Birth Statistics 2008). In these very low birthweight infants, there is increased incidence of non-verbal learning disabilities, behavioural disorders and an increased need for special educational assistance (Aylward 2002). In extremely low birthweight infants (birthweight below 1000g), approximately 10% exhibit cerebral palsy and 50% exhibit cognitive and behavioural deficits (Hack et al. 2000, Johnson et al. 2009). Children who escape cerebral palsy (CP) are at risk of motor impairments during their school years, while neuromotor abnormalities are the most frequent disability in ex-preterm children (Bracewell and Marlow 2002).

Pathology of brain injury in preterm infants

Brain injury in the preterm infant consists of multiple lesions, principally germinal matrix intraventricular haemorrhage (Fig. 7.1a), post-haemorrhagic hydrocephalus (Fig. 7.1b) and periventricular leukomalacia (PVL), which affects the white matter. White matter injury (WMI) is now the most important determinant of neurological morbidity observed in very low birthweight survivors.

Khwaja and Volpe (2008) described three major forms of WMI: (1) cystic PVL, in which focal necrosis is macroscopic and evolves to multiple cysts; (2) non-cystic PVL, in which the focal necrosis is microscopic and evolves primarily to glial scars and (3) diffuse white matter astrogliosis without focal necrosis, which may represent the mildest form of the spectrum of cerebral WMI. The cystic and non-cystic forms of PVL represent the two components of WMI. Cystic PVL is the focal necrosis component, which occurs deep in the cerebral white matter and where there is loss of all cellular elements (Fig. 7.2a and b). Non-cystic PVL is the diffuse and more superficial component, which occurs in the cerebral white matter with loss of pre-myelinating oligodendrocytes, astrogliosis and microglial infiltration (Khwaja and Volpe 2008).

When the focal necrotic component is large, subsequent cyst formation known as cystic PVL is readily visualised by cranial ultrasonography (Fig. 7.2). Formerly affecting around 8% of very low birthweight infants (Weindling et al. 1985), this lesion is now less common (around 1%–2%) because of improvements in neonatal intensive care management and

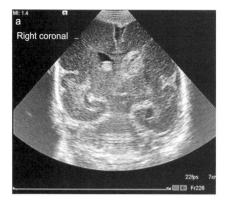
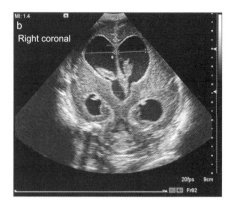

Fig. 7.1. Cranial ultrasound image from an infant born at 26 weeks' gestation. (a) On the first day after birth, the coronal image shows bilateral intraventricular haemorrhage with left parenchymal haemorrhagic infarction. (b) At 4 weeks of age, a repeat cranial ultrasound showed progressive dilatation of the ventricular system. The frontal index of the lateral ventricle measured 19mm on the right and 18mm on the left. The third ventricle measured 11mm. Cystic changes in the periventricular white matter on the left and early development of a porencephalic cyst are seen.

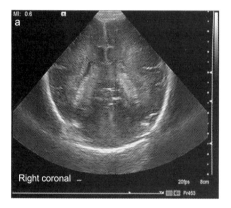
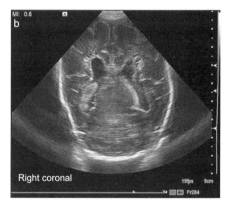

Fig. 7.2. Cranial ultrasound of an infant born at 29 weeks' gestation with prolonged rupture of membranes. (a) Image taken on the first day after birth, showing periventricular echogenicity and intraventricular haemorrhage. (b) At 3 weeks of age, the lateral ventricles are moderately dilated and have increased in size compared to the previous scan. The periventricular ischaemic change is now well established, showing changes consistent with cystic PVL. Extra-axial cerebrospinal fluid spaces are enlarged representing a reduction in brain volume.

accounts for only a small minority of PVL (van Haastert, I et al. 2011). More commonly, focal necroses are microscopic in size and evolve over several weeks to glial scars that are not readily seen by cranial ultrasonography. In recent years, the use of magnetic resonance imaging of the brain has provided significant insight into the pathology of these lesions.

Although controversy surrounds the principle initiating pathogenic factors in WMI, there is a strong argument for multiple insults, including hypoxic ischaemia and maternal intrauterine and/or fetal or neonatal infection. With the introduction of antenatal steroids, improved resuscitation techniques, better temperature control and surfactant therapy, preterm infants are now less likely to experience significant cardio-respiratory instability (see Chapter 11). There is no direct support for a causal relationship between hypoxic ischaemia and WMI in preterm infants, but there are important relevant observations. First, the cerebral vasculature of the very preterm infant is immature and differs from that of more mature infants (Malamateniou et al. 2006) and the anatomical distribution of injury appears to be in a watershed region of the brain (Wigglesworth et al. 1978), where the precursor cells for myelination, the pre-oligodendrocytes, appear to be susceptible to hypoxic ischaemia (Back et al. 2001). Second, clinical observations have related the lesion (cerebral WMI) to perinatal events expected to cause cerebral ischaemia, including marked hypocarbia (Greisen et al. 1987) and patent ductus arteriosus with retrograde cerebral diastolic flow (Shortland et al. 1990). Third, this disease of preterm birth is associated with maternal infection, which is sometimes sub-clinical (Wu & Colford, Jr. 2000). These observations suggest that a potentiating interaction between hypoxic ischaemia and infection/inflammation may now be the single most important cause of WMI.

Anatomical factors predisposing the preterm brain to injury

Several anatomical factors of the preterm brain increase its susceptibility to WMI, where myelin sheaths are generated by oligodendrocytes. Until 28 weeks' gestation, 90% of the total oligodendroglial population is comprised of 04-positive pre-oligodendrocytes. The remaining 10% being 01-positive cells (Back et al. 2001). Both cell types are susceptible to injurious mechanisms, as described later, but 04-positive cells are more vulnerable. The risk for PVL is related to the presence of these pre-oligodendrocytes in the periventricular white matter. Between 28 and 41 weeks, there is an increase in immature oligodendrocytes to nearly 50%, with concomitant increase in myelin sheaths. The decline in the incidence of PVL at around 32 weeks' gestation coincides with the onset of myelination in the periventricular white matter (Back et al. 2001) and presumably to the maturation of pre-oligodendrocytes to functioning oligodendrocytes. Maturational dependent factors therefore play a key role in the vulnerability of the cerebral white matter in preterm infants. Also noteworthy is the maturational dependent feature of microglial cells which play a central role in potentiating the interaction between systemic infection/inflammation and hypoxic ischaemia. Microglia are concentrated in the cerebral white matter and their concentration peaks at the time of greatest vulnerability to PVL, subsequently declining after 37 weeks' gestation (Billiards et al. 2006).

The focal and diffuse components of PVL appear to relate, in part, to the development of the vascular supply to cerebral white matter. This supply consists principally of short- and long-penetrating arteries. The focal component, with loss of all cellular elements, occurs principally in the end zones of these longer vessels. The distal fields of these vessels are not fully developed in the preterm infant and thus, decreases in cerebral blood flow in these areas would be expected to result in severe hypoxic-ischaemic injury. The diffuse component of PVL occurs principally in the distributions of (1) the border zones between the individual long-penetrating arteries and (2) the end zones of the short-penetrating arteries. These short-penetrating arteries do not develop fully until post-term. Thus, moderate hypoxic ischaemia would therefore be expected to result in a loss of pre-myelinating oligodendrocytes and microglial cells in this watershed zone.

Physiological factors predisposing the preterm brain to injury

Regional cerebral blood flow, measured by positron emission tomography in the cerebral white matter of surviving preterm infants with normal or near normal neurological outcomes, ranges from 1.6 to 3.0mL/100g/min (Altman et al. 1988). These flow values are markedly smaller than threshold values for viability in the adult human brain, that is, 10mL/100g/min (Powers et al. 1985). These remarkably low values in cerebral white matter are approximately 25% of those in cortical gray matter, a regional difference later confirmed in a study using single photon emission tomography (Borch and Greisen 1998). The very low values of volemic flow in cerebral white matter suggest that there is a minimal margin of safety for blood flow to cerebral white matter in such infants.

In our own studies, we have investigated cerebral oxygen delivery using electroencephalography (EEG) recordings and near-infrared spectroscopy (Young et al. 1982, Yoxall et al. 1995, Yoxall and Weindling 1998, Wardle et al. 2000, Kissack et al. 2004, 2005, Victor et al. 2006a). EEG recordings in very immature newborn infants, during the first 48 hours after birth, showed that EEG interburst intervals were prolonged only when mean blood pressure was below 23 mmHg (Victor et al. 2006a). EEG activity was normal (i.e. appropriate for gestational and postnatal age) despite low left and right ventricular cardiac outputs, suggesting that in preterm infants brain function was relatively protected from ischaemic injury (Victor et al. 2006b). Further evidence that factors operate to protect the preterm brain from injury are revealed by responses to hypocarbia. At low levels of blood carbon dioxide, brain metabolism (as demonstrated by brain electrical activity) slows down and cerebral fractional oxygen extraction increases (Victor et al. 2005). Both factors are brain protective.

Hypoxic ischaemia and preterm brain injury

The remainder of this chapter will focus on the two mechanisms of hypoxic ischaemia and infection/inflammation that cause PVL. They often operate together, apparently potentiating each other and are both important targets for strategies to prevent or ameliorate PVL.

The evidence for hypoxic ischaemia as a significant pathogenic mechanism is derived from animal models in which decreased cerebral blood flow leads to predominant WMI (Rice III et al. 1981, Young et al. 1982). Consequently, much of acute intensive care management focuses on the maintenance of an adequate blood and oxygen supply to the tissues, particularly the brain. Nonetheless, results from human studies are conflicting. For example, Dammann et al. (2002) and Logan et al. (2011) showed that systemic hypotension was not associated with cystic white matter injury as detected by cranial ultrasonography (Dammann et al. 2002, Young et al. 1982), whereas Chau et al. (2009) concluded that neonatal hypotension affected brain metabolic and microstructural development in preterm infants. Logan et al. (2011) and Alderliestein et al. (2014) showed that low blood pressure alone in preterm infants does not affect neurodevelopmental outcome at 18–24 months of age.

Despite the weak link between decreased cerebral oxygen delivery and WMI, cystic WMI is frequently detected in the watershed regions of the brain, supporting the hypothesis that hypoxic ischaemia is relevant for the pathogenesis of this condition. One reason why no link has been demonstrated between systemic hypotension and WMI may be that systemic hypotension is a poor marker of cerebral blood flow, due to factors such as cerebral auto-regulation and the ability for blood to be diverted to the brain from other organs (e.g. the skin, kidneys and gut). Under these circumstances, cardiac output is altered by shunting through the patent ductus arteriosus and patent foramen ovale in preterm infants and is therefore a poor estimate of cerebral blood flow. Accordingly, superior vena caval flow may be a better measure of cerebral blood flow and can be measured non-invasively using echocardiography (Kluckow and Evans 2000a, Moran et al. 2009). In this regard, low superior vena caval flow in the first hours after preterm birth is strongly associated with intraventricular haemorrhage (Kluckow and Evans 2000b) and persistently reduced flow, for the first 24 hours after birth, is significantly associated with death and abnormal developmental quotient in survivors (Hunt et al. 2004).

Maternal infection/inflammation and preterm brain injury

A number of epidemiological studies have shown an association between maternal/fetal infection and sonographically detectable WMI and cerebral palsy (Leviton et al. 1999, Wu and Colford, Jr. 2000). There is also evidence that the fetal immunological response is a more important risk factor than maternal inflammation (Dammann and Leviton 2000, Dammann et al. 2001). Raised levels of cytokines in neonatal blood and amniotic fluid as expressions of the humoral characteristics of the fetal immunological response have been associated with an increased incidence of WMI and cerebral palsy (Yoon et al. 1996, Wu and Colford, Jr. 2000, Yoon et al. 2000). A logistic regression model showed that high concentrations of cytokines in umbilical venous blood predicted brain injury ($p = 0.002$) with sensitivity of 60%, specificity of 78% and area under the ROC of 85% (Duggan et al. 2001). IL-6 -174 and -572 genotypes are associated with reduced volumes of deep grey matter (Reiman et al. 2009). However, despite several studies associating cytokines with brain injury, the precise role of cytokines in brain injury and repair is still unclear. It is also not clear, why some infants with elevated cord cytokine concentrations or maternal chorioamnionitis escape WMI, while others succumb (Kaukola et al. 2006).

In terms of causative agents, non-bacterial causes of fetal inflammation, including some viruses, for example, cytomegalovirus, rubella and others, are known to cross the human placenta, activate inflammatory pathways and increase concentrations of IL-6, IL-8 and TNF-alpha (Chou et al. 2006). Other viruses, such as herpes simplex virus and Epstein–Barr virus, have very little damaging effects on the developing embryo. Also, their incidence is relatively low, with only 2.5% of fetal and perinatal autopsies demonstrating evidence of any viral load (the vast majority being rubella) (Horn and Rose 1998).

Interaction of hypoxic ischaemia and maternal infection/inflammation

There is gathering evidence of a potentiating interaction between hypoxic ischaemia and infection/inflammation in causing WMI in preterm infants. Fetal and neonatal infection has been associated with persistent systemic hypotension and impaired cerebrovascular auto-regulation Yanowitz et al. 2002. Conversely hypoxic ischaemia, even in the absence of infection, causes systemic and cerebral elevation of microglia-derived vasoactive cytokines such as TNF-alpha and interleukin (IL-1beta) (Cheranov and Jaggar 2006).

In a previous study, Kadhim et al. (2001) described 19 infants with PVL and with asphyxia in the background. Although cytokine immune-reactivity was consistently detected in microglia, in patients superimposed with systemic fetal infections these levels were doubled. A further study of 61 preterm infants showed radiological evidence of WMI only in infants with a history of chorioamnionitis and concurrent placental perfusion defects (Redline et al. 2007).

Evidence of potentiation between infection/inflammation and ischaemia has also been shown in a number of animal studies in which pre-treatment with lipopolysaccharides at doses not sufficient to cause cerebral injury caused a sub-threshold hypoxic-ischaemic insult to elicit severe tissue damage (Girard et al. 2008a, Girard et al. 2008b). In rat models, the extent of cerebral infarction is also greatly enhanced following combined low dose endotoxin and a short period of hypoxic ischaemia, more so than exposure to either alone (Eklind et al. 2001).

In humans, a retrospective medical review by Yanowitz et al. (2004) showed that funisitis and fetal vasculitis were associated with hypotension and WMI. They also demonstrated an inverse relationship between IL-6 and mean blood pressure (Yanowitz et al. 2002). However, only Chau et al. (2009) have examined the relationship between neonatal hypotension, histopathological chorioamnionitis and abnormalities of brain metabolism and microstructure in preterm infants. They found that neonatal hypotension (odds ratio: 4 [95% CI: 1.4 – 11.5]) and not histopathological chorioamnionitis was the link to abnormal metabolic and microstructural brain development. Thus, this potentiating theory may be overvalued.

Hypoxic ischaemia and infection/inflammation, the two main initiating mechanisms, may act separately or in concert to activate two principal downstream mechanisms of excitotoxicity and free radical attack by reactive oxygen and nitrative attack. In this regard, the mechanisms underlying the maturation-dependent vulnerability of pre-oligodendrocytes has been addressed in both human and experimental studies in the preterm brain. It is proposed that microglia may play a central role in the generation of reactive oxygen and nitrative species and this role may be greater in response to combinations of ischaemia and infection/inflammation. A recent study of human PVL has shown a marked microgliosis in the diffuse component of PVL. It may therefore be that insults converge on the microglial cells to provoke a deleterious series of events, leading to secretion of toxic products, especially reactive oxygen and nitrative species, culminating in pre-oligodendroglial death (Khwaja & Volpe 2008).

Despite gathering evidence of the potentiating interaction between hypoxic ischaemia and maternal infection/inflammation, there is still no single study on the human preterm population which clearly demonstrates or refutes this relationship. Understanding the mechanisms of preterm brain injury and the complex interaction between hypoxic-ischaemia and fetal immunological response to maternal infection/inflammation, is fundamental for designing future treatment strategies.

REFERENCES

Alderliesten T, Lemmers PM, van Haastert IC et al. (2014) Hypotension in preterm neonates: Low blood pressure alone does not affect neurodevelopmental outcome. *J Pediatr* 164(5): 986–991. doi: http://dx.doi.org/10.1016/j.jpeds.2013.12.042

Altman DI, Powers WJ, Perlman JM, Herscovitch P, Volpe SL, Volpe JJ (1988) Cerebral blood flow requirement for brain viability in newborn infants is lower than in adults. *Ann Neurol* 24(2): 218–226. doi: http://dx.doi.org/10.1002/ana.410240208

Aylward GP (2002) Cognitive and neuropsychological outcomes: More than IQ scores. *Ment Retard Dev Dis Res Rev* 8(4): 234–240. doi: http://dx.doi.org/10.1002/mrdd.10043

Back SA, Luo NL, Borenstein NS, Levine JM, Volpe JJ, Kinney HC (2001) Late oligodendrocyte progenitors coincide with the developmental window of vulnerability for human perinatal white matter injury. *J Neurosci* 21(4): 1302–1312.

Billiards SS, Haynes RL, Folkerth RD et al. (2006) Development of microglia in the cerebral white matter of the human fetus and infant. *J Comp Neurol* 497(2): 199–208. doi: http://dx.doi.org/10.1002/cne.20991

Borch K, Greisen G (1998) Blood flow distribution in the normal human preterm brain. *Pediatr Res* 43(1): 28–33. doi: http://dx.doi.org/10.1203/00006450-199801000-00005

Bracewell M, Marlow N (2002) Patterns of motor disability in very preterm children. *Ment Retard Dev Dis Res Rev* 8(4): 241–248. doi: http://dx.doi.org/10.1002/mrdd.10049

Chau V, Poskitt KJ, McFadden DE et al. (2009) Effect of chorioamnionitis on brain development and injury in premature newborns. *Ann Neurol* 66(2): 155–164. doi: http://dx.doi.org/10.1002/ana.21713

Cheranov SY, Jaggar JH (2006) TNF-alpha dilates cerebral arteries via NAD(P)H oxidase-dependent Ca2+ spark activation. *Am J Physiol: Cell Physiol* 290(4): C964–C971. Epub 2005 Nov 2. doi: http://dx.doi.org/10.1152/ajpcell.00499.2005

Chou D, Ma Y, Zhang J, McGrath C, Parry S (2006) Cytomegalovirus infection of trophoblast cells elicits an inflammatory response: A possible mechanism of placental dysfunction. *Am J Obst Gynecol* 194(2): 535–541. doi: http://dx.doi.org/10.1016/j.ajog.2005.07.073

Dammann O, Allred EN, Kuban KC et al. (2002) Systemic hypotension and white-matter damage in preterm infants. *Dev Med Child Neurol* 44(2): 82–90. doi: http://dx.doi.org/10.1111/j.1469-8749.2002.tb00292.x

Dammann O, Durum S, Leviton A (2001) Do white cells matter in white matter damage? *Trends Neurosci* 24(6): 320–324. doi: http://dx.doi.org/10.1016/s0166-2236(00)01811-7

Dammann O, Leviton A (2000) Role of the fetus in perinatal infection and neonatal brain damage. *Curr Opin Pediatr* 12(2): 99–104. doi: http://dx.doi.org/10.1097/00008480-200004000-00002

Duggan PJ, Maalouf EF, Watts TL et al. (2001) Intrauterine T-cell activation and increased proinflammatory cytokine concentrations in preterm infants with cerebral lesions. *Lancet* 358(9294): 1699–1700. doi: http://dx.doi.org/10.1016/s0140-6736(01)06723-x

Eklind S, Mallard C, Leverin AL et al. (2001) Bacterial endotoxin sensitizes the immature brain to hypoxic--ischaemic injury. *Eur J Neurosci* 13(6): 1101–1106. doi: http://dx.doi.org/10.1046/j.0953-816x.2001.01474.x

Girard S, Kadhim H, Larouche A, Roy M, Gobeil F, Sebire G (2008a) Pro-inflammatory disequilibrium of the IL-1 beta/IL-1ra ratio in an experimental model of perinatal brain damages induced by lipopolysaccharide and hypoxia-ischemia. *Cytokine* 43(1): 54–62. doi: http://dx.doi.org/10.1016/j.cyto.2008.04.007

Girard S, Larouche A, Kadhim H, Rola-Pleszczynski M, Gobeil F, Sebire G (2008b) Lipopolysaccharide and hypoxia/ischemia induced IL-2 expression by microglia in neonatal brain. *Neuroreport* 19(10): 997–1002. doi: http://dx.doi.org/10.1097/wnr.0b013e3283036e88

Greisen G, Munck H, Lou H (1987) Severe hypocarbia in preterm infants and neurodevelopmental deficit. *Acta Paediatr Scand* 76(3): 401–404. doi: http://dx.doi.org/10.1111/j.1651-2227.1987.tb10489.x

Hack M, Wilson-Costello D, Friedman H, Taylor GH, Schluchter M, Fanaroff AA (2000) Neurodevelopment and predictors of outcomes of children with birth weights of less than 1000 g: 1992–1995. *Arch Pediatr Adolesc Med* 154(7): 725–731. doi: http://dx.doi.org/10.1001/archpedi.154.7.725

Horn LC, Rose I (1998) Placental and fetal pathology in intrauterine viral infections. *Intervirol* 41(4–5): 219–225. doi: http://dx.doi.org/10.1159/000024940

Hunt RW, Evans N, Rieger I, Kluckow M (2004) Low superior vena caval flow and neurodevelopment at 3 years in very preterm infants. *J Pediatr* 145(5): 588–592. doi: http://dx.doi.org/10.1016/j.jpeds.2004.06.056

Johnson S, Hennessy EM, Smith R, Trikic R, Wolke D, Marlow N (2009) Academic attainment and special educational needs in extremely preterm children at 11 years of age: The EPICure Study. *Arch Dis Child* 94(4): F283–F289. doi: http://dx.doi.org/10.1136/adc.2008.152793

Kadhim H, Tabarki B, Verellen G, De Prez C, Rona AM, Sébire G (2001) Inflammatory cytokines in the pathogenesis of periventricular leukomalacia. *Neurology* 56(10): 1278–1284. doi: http://dx.doi.org/10.1212/wnl.56.10.1278

Kaukola T, Herva R, Perhomaa M et al. (2006) Population cohort associating chorioamnionitis, cord inflammatory cytokines and neurologic outcome in very preterm, extremely low birth weight infants. *Pediatr Res* 59(3): 478–483. doi: http://dx.doi.org/10.1203/01.pdr.0000182596.66175.ee

Khwaja O, Volpe JJ (2008) Pathogenesis of cerebral white matter injury of prematurity. *Arch Dis Child Fetal Neonatal Ed* 93(2): F153–F161. doi: http://dx.doi.org/10.1136/adc.2006.108837

Kissack CM, Garr R, Wardle SP, Weindling AM (2004) Cerebral fractional oxygen extraction in very low birth weight infants is high when there is low left ventricular output and hypocarbia but is unaffected by hypotension. *Pediatr Res* 55(3): 400–405. doi: http://dx.doi.org/10.1203/01.pdr.0000111288.87002.3a

Kissack CM, Garr R, Wardle SP et al. (2005) Cerebral fractional oxygen extraction is inversely correlated with oxygen delivery in the sick, newborn, preterm infant. *J Cereb Blood Flow Metab* 25(5): 545–553. doi: http://dx.doi.org/10.1038/sj.jcbfm.9600046

Kluckow M, Evans N (2000a) Superior vena cava flow in newborn infants: A novel marker of systemic blood flow. *Arch Dis Child Fetal Neonatal Ed* 82(3): F182–F187. doi: http://dx.doi.org/10.1136/fn.82.3.f182

Kluckow M, Evans N (2000b) Low superior vena cava flow and intraventricular haemorrhage in preterm infants. *Arch Dis Child Fetal Neonatal Ed* 82(3): F188–F194. doi: http://dx.doi.org/10.1136/fn.82.3.f188

Leviton A, Paneth N, Reuss ML et al. (1999) Maternal infection, fetal inflammatory response, and brain damage in very low birth weight infants. Developmental Epidemiology Network Investigators. *Pediatr Res* 46(5): 566–575. doi: http://dx.doi.org/10.1203/00006450-199911000-00013

Logan JW, O'Shea TM, Allred EN et al. (2011) ELGAN study investigators. Early postnatal hypotension is not associated with indicators of white matter damage or cerebral palsy in extremely low gestational age newborns. *J Perinatol* 31(8): 524–534. doi: http://dx.doi.org/10.1038/jp.2010.201

Malamateniou C, Counsell SJ, Allsop JM et al. (2006) The effect of preterm birth on neonatal cerebral vasculature studied with magnetic resonance angiography at 3 Tesla. *Neuroimage* 32(3): 1050–1059. doi: http://dx.doi.org/10.1016/j.neuroimage.2006.05.051

Moran M, Miletin J, Pichova K, Dempsey EM (2009) Cerebral tissue oxygenation index and superior vena cava blood flow in the very low birth weight infant. *Acta Paediatr* 98(1): 43–46. doi: http://dx.doi.org/10.1111/j.1651-2227.2008.01006.x

Office of National Statistics, Birth Statistics 2008. Review of the National Statistician on Births and Patterns of Family Building in England and Wales 2008. ONS London, Series FM1 No 37:1-110.

Powers WJ, Grubb RL, Jr., Darriet D, Raichle ME (1985) Cerebral blood flow and cerebral metabolic rate of oxygen requirements for cerebral function and viability in humans. *J Cereb Blood Flow Metab* 5(4): 600–608. doi: http://dx.doi.org/10.1038/jcbfm.1985.89

Redline RW, Minich N, Taylor HG, Hack M (2007) Placental lesions as predictors of cerebral palsy and abnormal neurocognitive function at school age in extremely low birth weight infants (<1 kg). *Pediatr Dev Pathol* 10(4): 282–292. doi: http://dx.doi.org/10.2350/06-12-0203.1

Reiman M, Parkkola R, Lapinleimu H, Lehtonen L, Haataja L (2009) Interleukin-6 -174 and -572 genotypes and the volume of deep gray matter in preterm infants. *Pediatr Res* 65(1): 90–96. doi: http://dx.doi.org/10.1203/pdr.0b013e31818bbfac

Rice JE, III, Vannucci RC, Brierley JB (1981) The influence of immaturity on hypoxic-ischemic brain damage in the rat. *Ann Neurol* 9(2): 131–141. doi: http://dx.doi.org/10.1002/ana.410090206

Shortland DB, Gibson NA, Levene MI, Archer LN, Evans DH, Shaw DE (1990) Patent ductus arteriosus and cerebral circulation in preterm infants. *Dev Med Child Neurol* 32(5): 386–393. doi: http://dx.doi.org/10.1111/j.1469-8749.1990.tb16957.x

van Haastert IC, Groenendaal F, Uiterwaal CS et al. (2011) Decreasing incidence and severity of cerebral palsy in prematurely born children. *J Pediatr* 159(1): 86–91. doi: http://dx.doi.org/10.1016/j.jpeds.2010.12.053

Victor S, Appleton RE, Beirne M, Marson AG, Weindling AM (2005) Effect of carbon dioxide on background cerebral electrical activity and fractional oxygen extraction in very low birth weight infants just after birth. *Pediatr Res* 58(3): 579–585. doi: http://dx.doi.org/10.1203/01.pdr.0000169402.13435.09

Victor S, Marson AG, Appleton RE, Beirne M, Weindling AM (2006a) Relationship between blood pressure, cerebral electrical activity, cerebral fractional oxygen extraction, and peripheral blood flow in very low birth weight newborn infants. *Pediatr Res* 59(2): 314–319. doi: http://dx.doi.org/10.1203/01.pdr.0000199525.08615.1f

Victor S, Appleton RE, Beirne M, Marson AG, Weindling AM (2006b) The relationship between cardiac output, cerebral electrical activity, cerebral fractional oxygen extraction and peripheral blood flow in premature newborn infants. *Pediatr Res* 60(4): 456–460. doi: http://dx.doi.org/10.1203/01.pdr.0000238379.67720.19

Wardle SP, Yoxall CW, Weindling AM (2000) Determinants of cerebral fractional oxygen extraction using near infrared spectroscopy in preterm neonates. *J Cereb Blood Flow Metab* 20(2): 272–279. doi: http://dx.doi.org/10.1097/00004647-200002000-00008

Weindling AM, Rochefort MJ, Calvert SA, Fok TF, Wilkinson A (1985) Development of cerebral palsy after ultrasonographic detection of periventricular cysts in the newborn. *Dev Med Child Neurol* 27(6): 800–806. doi: http://dx.doi.org/10.1111/j.1469-8749.1985.tb03805.x

Wigglesworth JS, Pape KE, Wigglesworth JS, Pape KE (1978) An integrated model for haemorrhagic and ischaemic lesions in the newborn brain. *Early Hum Dev* 2(2): 179–199. doi: http://dx.doi.org/10.1016/0378-3782(78)90010-5

Wu YW, Colford JM Jr. (2000) Chorioamnionitis as a risk factor for cerebral palsy: A meta-analysis. *JAMA* 284(11): 1417–1424. doi: http://dx.doi.org/10.1001/jama.284.11.1417

Yanowitz TD, Baker RW, Roberts JM, Brozanski BS (2004) Low blood pressure among very-low-birth-weight infants with fetal vessel inflammation. *J Perinatol* 24(5): 299–304. doi: http://dx.doi.org/10.1038/sj.jp.7211091

Yanowitz TD, Jordan JA, Gilmour CH et al. (2002) Hemodynamic disturbances in premature infants born after chorioamnionitis: Association with cord blood cytokine concentrations. *Pediatr Res* 51(3): 310–316. doi: http://dx.doi.org/10.1203/00006450-200203000-00008

Yoon BH, Romero R, Park JS et al. (2000) Fetal exposure to an intra-amniotic inflammation and the development of cerebral palsy at the age of three years. *Am J Obstet Gynecol* 182(3): 675–681. doi: http://dx.doi.org/10.1067/mob.2000.104207

Yoon BH, Romero R, Yang SH et al. (1996) Interleukin-6 concentrations in umbilical cord plasma are elevated in neonates with white matter lesions associated with periventricular leukomalacia. *Am J Obstet Gynecol* 174(5): 1433–1440. doi: http://dx.doi.org/10.1016/s0002-9378(96)70585-9

Young RS, Hernandez MJ, Yagel SK (1982) Selective reduction of blood flow to white matter during hypotension in newborn dogs: A possible mechanism of periventricular leukomalacia. *Ann Neurol* 12(5): 445–448. doi: http://dx.doi.org/10.1002/ana.410120506

Yoxall CW, Weindling AM (1998) Measurement of cerebral oxygen consumption in the human neonate using near infrared spectroscopy: Cerebral oxygen consumption increases with advancing gestational age. *Pediatr Res* 44(3): 283–290. doi: http://dx.doi.org/10.1203/00006450-199809000-00004

8
IN UTERO IMAGING OF THE HUMAN PLACENTA

Emma Ingram and Ed Johnstone

Ultrasound imaging

Ultrasound examination was introduced into obstetric practice in 1978 and has become an integral part of fetal anomaly screening. Sonography allows accurate pregnancy dating, identification of multiple pregnancies and fetal anomalies (Roberts and Thilaganathan 2007). Yet, it is the use of ultrasound and Doppler techniques to identify and monitor pregnancies at risk of growth restriction which has become increasingly valuable (Turan et al. 2008).

Fetal growth can be monitored by estimation of fetal weight and growth velocity using serial measures of head, abdominal circumference and femur length (March et al. 2012). Since the majority of fetal growth disorders are secondary to placental disease, it is the placenta and its associated blood flow which has become prominent in screening and management of these compromised pregnancies (Sibley et al. 2005).

The advantage of ultrasound over other imaging modalities is its relative safety, affordability and capacity to produce real-time images. As ultrasound technology advances, new modalities such as 3D and 4D imaging may provide added benefit, but so far these techniques have failed to alter routine antenatal sonography.

Irrespective of ultrasound modality, image quality can be significantly affected by fetal position, artefact (created by air–water interface) and maternal habitus. These disadvantages, coupled with the functional capacity of alternative imaging techniques such as magnetic resonance imaging (MRI), may provide eventual impetus for the adoption of more costly imaging techniques.

Structural imaging of the human placenta

Ideally, a healthy placenta should have a discoid shape, with central cord insertion and a homogenous appearance on ultrasound. Using conventional 2D ultrasound, it is possible to measure placental size in three dimensions, identify structural abnormalities and classify placental maturation (Grannum grading) dependent on the presence and location of calcification (Grannum et al. 1979).

Sonographic identification of accelerated placental maturity (Grannum III) before 36 weeks' gestation is associated with pregnancy-induced hypertension, fetal growth restriction (FGR) and fetal distress in labour, all of which contribute to an increased risk of morbidity and mortality (McKenna et al. 2005). However, studies have suggested this method, although potentially valuable, lacks objectivity, precision and reproducibility (Sau et al. 2004).

Eccentric cord insertion is also associated with low birthweight infants, preterm birth and intrapartum complications (Liu et al. 2002). With optimal development, the placental vasculature is thought to radiate symmetrically from a central insertion point (Yampolsky et al. 2009). The accurate assessment of cord insertion using ultrasound requires the entire placental length to be captured in a single image and is, therefore, more difficult in late gestation. The sensitivity and specificity of diagnosing non-central cord insertion is improved with the addition of the colour and power Doppler techniques (Pretorius et al. 1996).

For many years, the depth and length of the placenta has been related to pregnancy success, with thicker placentas of smaller diameter associated more frequently with complications, secondary to placental insufficiency (Salafia et al. 2006). Although uncertain, this more globular shape is postulated to be a poor adaptive response to increased placental proficiency by exaggerating villus vascularity (Todros et al. 1999). Two-dimensional ultrasound assessments of placental size seem to confirm this suggestion. In a high-risk population, a placental thickness greater than 4cm (or 50% of the placental diameter) or a placental diameter of less than 10cm is associated with adverse perinatal outcomes, particularly FGR (Fisteag-Kiprono et al. 2006, Toal ct al. 2008). Nevertheless, these cut-offs are largely historical and other studies of placental diameter in predicting FGR at delivery have been confounded by an eccentric cord (Hoddick et al. 1985, Costantini et al. 2012). Undoubtedly, confirmation of a reference range of sonographically measured placental size is required before it can be used as a screening tool in low-risk pregnancies.

An alternative measure of placental insufficiency may be placental volume, using a 3D ultrasound technique termed 'virtual organ computer aided analysis' (VOCAL). There is evidence that sonographic differences in placental volume are detectable as early as the first trimester and can predict the development of issues subsequent to placental dysfunction (Hafner et al. 1998, Rizzo et al. 2008). This technique has good inter- and intra-observer reproducibility, but its sensitivity is dependent on early pathophysiological diagnosis of placental disease (Deurloo et al. 2007). Volume reductions in pregnancies affected by placental insufficiency should be more pronounced by the third trimester. However, as with 2D measurements, difficulty in determining entire placental volumes in late gestation currently limits its use as a diagnostic tool (Azpurua et al. 2010).

In addition to these gross volumetric determinations, 3D surface-rendering techniques may offer a new visual experience in examining the human placenta. The near photographic depiction of the placental surface may aid detection of placental abnormalities, but this technique is in its infancy, with limited studies on sensitivity and reproducibility to date.

Utero-placental blood flow
More functional estimations of placental blood flow can be measured using 2D Doppler ultrasound. The Doppler signal is depicted in four parameters: (1) pulsatility index (2) resistance (3) index, systolic/diastolic ratio and, for certain vessels, (4) peak systolic volume, which defines blood flow throughout the cardiac cycle. These measures are dependent on

fetal size and gestation and can be used as a means of screening for potential pregnancy complications and evidence of fetal compromise. Because of their broad reference range, minor increases in a single ultrasound examination may be easily masked. Consequently, serial Doppler measurements are beneficial in identifying trends in blood flow, while comparisons between vessels can also yield useful information as to the degree of fetal compensation and mismatch in placental perfusion.

In the non-pregnant state, the uterine artery Doppler waveform is characterised by an early diastolic notch and high resistance (Kalache and Duckelmann 2012). Upon placentation, the calibre of these arteries is increased, generating vessels of high flow, low resistance and an absent notch, optimising uterine blood flow (Fig. 8.1a). When present, the persistence of high resistance can be viewed as a proxy for abnormal placentation and can be found in pre-eclampsia and FGR (Fig. 8.1a). Several studies have shown that uterine artery Doppler examination in the first and second trimester are sensitive in identifying patients at risk of developing early onset pre-eclampsia and to a lesser extent FGR (Sciscione and Hayes 2009, Meler et al. 2010), most notably in high-risk women (i.e. those with a history of chronic hypertension, pre-eclampsia, prior FGR or stillbirth). In these patients, abnormal assessments may warrant increased antenatal surveillance. Despite these benefits, the limited predictive value of uterine Doppler in a low-risk obstetric cohort, alongside the lack of available interventions, means that routine uterine artery Doppler is currently not endorsed for regular antenatal care (Alfirevic et al. 2010).

As an adjunct to 2D ultrasound, colour-flow Doppler has allowed real-time visualisation of jets of maternal blood emerging from the uterine spiral arteries (Collins et al. 2012). This method may aid in understanding abnormal placentation by measuring the actual pathology at the utero-placental interface, rather than the uterine artery as an 'upstream' surrogate. Although it was envisaged that characterisation of these jets would one day benefit screening for adverse pregnancies, this has yet to be realised. In the meantime, alternative approaches to visualising and reconstructing the placental vasculature have shown promise. Three-dimensional power Doppler (Fig. 8.1b) has shown recent success in visualising reduced placental vascularity and impaired vascular budding in FGR pregnancies (Hata et al. 2011). Likewise, this technique has been applied to identifying vasa praevia and visualising anastomoses in monochorionic twins (Lee et al. 2000, Welsh et al. 2001).

Three-dimensional Doppler techniques, used to quantify blood flow in other organs, have also been applied to the human placenta, in a practice termed 'placental vascular biopsy' (Hata et al. 2011). This technique produces three parameters: a vascularisation index, flow index and vascular flow index, combining information concerning vessel presence and blood flow. Attempts to establish a placental reference range have shown little consistency, with vascular models demonstrating that measures are susceptible to changes in gain settings, commonly adjusted in sonographic practice. Despite inconsistencies, vascular flow index has been shown to be lower in FGR pregnancies, particularly those with reduced pregnancy-associated plasma protein A (PAPPA), and vascularisation index has a reported linear relationship with birthweight (Guiot et al. 2008, Rizzo et al. 2009, Bozkurt et al. 2010). This notwithstanding, strong disagreement in their application to the placenta abounds and further study is required.

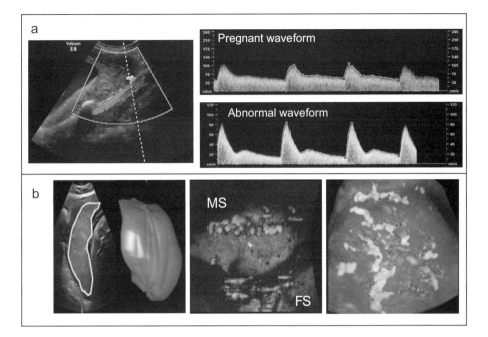

Fig. 8.1. Ultrasound investigations of the utero-placenta. (a) Identification and Doppler waveform of the uterine artery. Abnormal placentation characterised by elevated resistance and retained early diastolic notch. (b) 3D ultrasound showing volume determination of the placenta and power Doppler rendering of placental blood flow on the placental chorionic (fetal side FS) and basal plate (maternal side MS). A colour version of this figure can be seen in the plate section at the end of the book.

Feto-placental blood flow

As with uterine arteries, Doppler ultrasound assessments of umbilical vessels are commonly used as surrogates for downstream resistance in the feto-placental vasculature. Sequential changes in these vessels are seen in severe FGR, progressing from reduced to absent and ultimately reversed umbilical flow during fetal ventricular diastole (Baschat et al. 2000). Pathological studies have shown increased impedance within umbilical arteries evident when at least 60% of the placental vasculature is obliterated. While an abnormal Doppler waveform is strongly associated with poor perinatal outcome and high mortality (Kalache and Duckelmann 2012), a normal waveform (in contrast) is rarely associated with signifi-cant morbidity, even in fetuses of low gestational weight. Thus, as with uterine artery assessments, the clinical use of umbilical Doppler is recommended in the prevention of perinatal deaths in high-risk pregnancies only (Alfirevic et al. 2010).

While an increased umbilical artery resistance may be indicative to expedite delivery, cases with extreme prematurity, associated with FGR, are more difficult to manage. In these complex cases, clinicians can deploy Doppler studies of additional fetal vessels to accurately assess the risk of in utero death. Such vessels include the middle cerebral artery (MCA) and ductus venosus.

Under chronic fetal oxygen deprivation and under-nutrition, it is recognised that the fetal circulation compensates with redistribution of blood to essential organs, most notably the heart, adrenals and brain. This diversion is often termed 'brain-sparing' and is associated with increased resistance in the umbilical artery and ductus venosus and reduced resistance in the MCA. Although low MCA pulsatility index (PI) has predictive value for perinatal mortality, subsequent restoration in MCA-peak systolic volume (PSV) and PI maybe a sign of impending fetal demise (Simanaviciute and Gudmundsson 2006). As with other Doppler investigations, repeated observations provide more clinical information than a single examination alone (Johnson et al. 2001) and in this instance, care should be taken to minimise abdominal pressure during monitoring, as fetal head compression is associated with alterations in intra-cranial arterial waveforms. Other ultrasound findings, which may accompany this redistribution of fetal blood, include decreased amniotic fluid and increased bowel echogenicity.

Within the fetal circulation, the ductus venosus shunts a proportion of oxygenated blood from the umbilical vein to the inferior vena cava at its inlet to the heart. A typical waveform results, demonstrating two peaks: one generated by ventricular contraction and the other an atrial contraction (or 'a wave'). With mounting placental insufficiency, the proportion of shunted blood increases, leading to an elevation in DV resistance and eventual loss and reversal of the 'a wave' (Baschat 2010). These changes in DV waveform, which can be viewed as fetal hemodynamic decompensation (akin to right heart failure) also portent to fetal demise. The absence or reversal of the a-wave predicts fetal acidosis with 65% sensitivity and 95% specificity (Baschat et al. 2003). Analysis of DV Doppler waveform is often used to supplement umbilical artery and MCA Doppler readings, in defining judicious timing of delivery.

Contemporary placental imaging

As evident, current methods of imaging the human placenta and investigating high-risk pregnancies are concentrated on ultrasound estimations of placental size, structure, fetal biometry and Doppler studies. Although ultrasound has proven invaluable in monitoring pregnancies, superior methods for predicting placenta malfunction are desirable, to evaluate and optimise treatment. Ideally, non-invasive measures of placental structure, as well as function (i.e. perfusion and oxygenation), may aid in these assessments. Magnetic resonance imaging (MRI) has the ability to assess placental structure and function and therefore holds potential in providing additional antenatal information for diagnosing and monitoring compromised pregnancies.

Magnetic resonance imaging and the placenta

In general, the placenta is an ideal organ to study with MRI, because of its relative immobility, large blood volume and absence of tissue–air interfaces, which generate artefact. MRI has been used extensively in pregnancy with no adverse maternal or fetal effects. Nevertheless, in order to maximise safety and comfort, certain considerations and limitations are required. The pregnant woman should be scanned on a lateral tilt to reduce aorto-caval compression and many advocate entering the bore feet-first to reduce claustrophobia and anxiety. While an MRI poses no radiation risk, the process does generate heat and noise, as studied in animal and human models. Heat deposition from radio-frequency magnetic fields should be limited by low specific absorption rate (SAR) modes, which prevent potential teratogenic effects. Changing gradient fields creates acoustic noise, as the receiver coils impact on the mountings. Although the noise reaching the fetal cochlear is attenuated by the maternal abdomen and amniotic fluid, it is important to ensure that direct coupling (vibration) between the mother's body and bed is minimised.

So far the use of placental specific MRI has been limited to an adjunct to ultrasound, in defining depth of invasion in the morbidly adherent placenta. As a research tool, MRI has only recently found favour in the study of placental structure and function. In general, the appearance of the normal healthy placenta on MRI is relatively homogenous, with a low signal intensity on T1-weighted images and high signal intensity on T2-weighted equivalents. Although placental heterogeneities are observed with increasing gestation, these may be exaggerated in complicated pregnancies, thought to correspond to regions of infarct, necrosis and fibrosis. These heterogeneities have been demonstrated by ultrasound and MRI. For such pathologies, signal intensities have been correlated with postnatal histology (Linduska et al. 2009) and FGR severity (Damodaram et al. 2010).

From MRI, placenta volume can be measured using a set of multi-slice images. This process is unaffected by ultrasound limitations, such as maternal habitus, amniotic fluid, fetal position and gestational age. Against amniotic fluid, the boundary of the placenta is exceptionally clear; although less so with the uterine wall, this can be surmised from its geometry (Fig. 8.2). As with other modalities, there is a significant association between placental volume and birthweight (Heinonen et al. 2001), but not maternal factors such as age, body mass index and smoking. Although early MRI studies suggested that placental volume is generally lower in growth restricted pregnancies, this failed to fall beyond the confidence limits of the normal population (Baker et al. 1995). However, with more robust

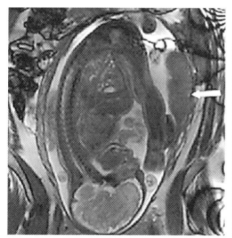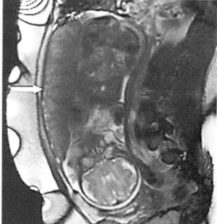

Fig. 8.2. MRI structural fetal images (sagittal [left], coronal [right], T2 HASTE sequence) used to localise placental position. These images demonstrate a cephalic fetal presentation with anterior placenta (arrowed). The fetal brain, spinal cord and abdominal organs are clearly identified.

definitions of FGR, using individualised birthweight ratios (IBRs) and abnormal Doppler observations, distinctions in volume have now been achieved (Derwig et al. 2011).

Histology has shown the normal placenta increases in villus surface area with maturation, while the proportion of blood remains relatively unchanged. MRI relaxation times are measureable parameters that may reflect these finer changes in tissue morphology. Longitudinal (T1) and transverse relaxation times (T2) of the placenta decrease with gestation and are further reduced in pregnancies complicated by growth restriction (Gowland et al. 1998). At 1.5Tesla, placental T1 and T2 relaxation times in healthy pregnancies have shown a linear relationship with gestation, decreasing by 20.2ms and 2.4ms per week respectively (Wright et al. 2011). These times are shorter than corresponding values for blood at the same field strength, implying that the villus surface area, rather than blood per se, has the greater influence. One magnetic resonance magnetisation study, estimating the vascular to non-vascular content of the placenta, added weight to this theory (Ong et al. 2004), but arguably verification has been hindered by mismatches in time of delivery and scan (Wright et al. 2011).

Magnetic resonance imaging of placental perfusion
Perfusion can be measured with MRI by multiple techniques. Early studies of placental perfusion were performed with gadolinium as a contrast agent, given for other clinical reasons (Marcos et al. 1997). In these rudimentary studies, the placenta showed a lobular appearance, becoming confluent at the myometrial interface. Safety concerns regarding fetal exposure to contrast cavitation have meant this method is contraindicated. The rate of clearance of contrast from the amniotic fluid is unknown and with its continual ingestion by the fetus, toxicity could also accumulate. Alternative, non-contrast methods for the determination placental perfusion have been applied, namely arterial spin labelling (ASL), flow sensitive alternating inversion recovery ASL (FAIR-ASL) and intravoxel incoherent motion (IVIM).

In ASL, magnetically labelled water is used for intrinsic contrast. A variation of this technique, FAIR-ASL, has been adapted for multi-directional blood flow within the placenta (Gowland et al. 1998). Using FAIR-ASL, the average perfusion rate of the placenta was found to be 176ml/100g/min, which, based on past knowledge, suggests an overestimation (Francis et al. 1998). Now proposed as an estimate of blood within a tissue, rather than classic perfusion, FAIR-ASL may still offer clinical relevance. The ability to determine FGR using FAIR was suggested by Derwig et al. (2013). They demonstrated that small for gestational age fetuses had significantly reduced FAIR-derived perfusion at 24–29 weeks' gestation than those of appropriate size. With possible use in high-risk pregnancies, this technique has so far failed to improve upon uterine artery Doppler sensitivity in small for gestational age prediction (Derwig et al. 2013).

IVIM was initially devised for measuring perfusion in capillary networks using diffusion-weighted MRI. Water moving in such networks is modelled as a fraction of rapid voxel diffusion. The sequence is sensitive to blood moving in different directions and velocities. It is particularly effective in high flow regions. Initial studies averaged the moving blood fraction within the healthy placenta to be 26%, which reduces with gestation by 0.6% per week (Moore et al. 2000). Using this technique, several functional areas of the placenta have been determined, with highest flow defined in the basal plate. Two studies have reported a reduction in perfusion using IVIM in pregnancies affected by early onset preeclampsia and FGR (Derwig et al. 2013, Sohlberg et al. 2014).

Imaging of placental oxygenation

There is limited information about the oxygen environment of the placenta, with the majority coming from invasive procedures in early pregnancy (Jauniaux et al. 2001). MRI has the capability of providing non-invasive measures of placental oxygenation, which may prove effective in determining a placenta failing to meet its fetal requirements. With MRI, baseline oxygenation cannot be measured. However, blood-oxygen-level-dependent contrast imaging (BOLD) and oxygen-enhanced MRI (OE-MRI) can determine functional changes, using inspired oxygen as an endogenous contrast.

BOLD quantifies oxygen saturation within tissues due to the different magnetic properties of haemoglobin and deoxyhaemoglobin. Shorter T2* times, generated by paramagnetic deoxyhaemoglobin, produce measurable signal loss in areas of reduced oxygen saturation. Changes in saturation are calculated by subtraction of the BOLD signal produced under air from that of hyperoxia. The fetal aspect of the placenta demonstrates significant changes in BOLD with hyperoxia, due to its relative hypoxic nature, yet the maternal aspect remains largely unresponsive because of already highly saturated haemoglobin (Sørensen et al. 2013). While BOLD signal changes are reproducible in multiple slices and correlate closely with blood measures of oxygen saturation, this technique is dependent on other variables, including the haemoglobin concentration, haematocrit, blood flow and blood volume. Current observations suggest that fetal brain oxygenation fails to increase in response to maternal hyperoxia and that the absence of changes in the fetal brain may hold relevance in informing efficacy of maternal oxygen therapy to avert fetal morbidity/mortality (Huen et al. 2014).

Oxygen-enhanced MRI is a surrogate measure of the partial pressure of oxygen within tissues. Under hyperoxia, an increased proportion of oxygen molecules is dissolved

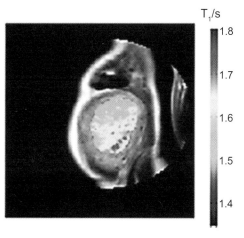

T_1/s

1.8

1.7

1.6

1.5

1.4

Fig. 8.3. Placental MRI map showing sensitivity to oxygen saturation (PO_2). T1-weighted image obtained in an in-plane view superimposed on a T2-weighted structural image. A colour version of this figure can be seen in the plate section at the end of the book.

within blood plasma. The close proximity of the paramagnetic oxygen to surrounding water generates dipolar interactions with hydrogen protons, decreasing T1 relaxation times (Fig. 8.3). Placental studies using OE-MRI demonstrate increased R1 (1/T1) times with increasing inspired oxygen concentrations. However, this positive change in R1 declines with gestational age (Huen et al. 2013). This may reflect lower fetal haemoglobin saturation, due to increasing demand on the maturing placenta, but, notably, changes in R1 between normal and compromised pregnancies have yet to be established.

Magnetic resonance spectroscopy

As an alternative to MRI, it is possible to estimate concentrations of specific metabolites by proton magnetic resonance spectroscopy (1H-MRS). As with MRI, in MRS protons are excited by radiofrequencies with local chemical structures determining resonant frequencies. This is known as the 'chemical shift'. The output is a frequency spectrum with the contributions of specific metabolites appearing as individual peaks, the area under each peak representing the number of protons and hence concentration of metabolites (Story et al. 2011).

In pregnancy, 1H-MRS is a research tool with exciting possibilities. Cell turnover within the healthy fetal brain creates a choline peak and N-acetylaspartate (NAA) peak, a derivative of aspartic acid. These increase with advancing gestation and neuronal development. A reduction in the NAA/choline ratio has been demonstrated in the fetal brain in infants with FGR (Story et al. 2011). Using this principal, spectroscopy of the placenta could be used to demonstrate the reduction in cell-turnover and increase in apoptosis seen in placentas from FGR pregnancies (Heazell et al. 2008). Cetin and Alvino (2009) suggest that such alterations in placental metabolism may precede the onset of placental and fetal hypoxia in affected pregnancies. Early studies into placental spectroscopy have demonstrated a severe attenuation or absence of detectable choline in placentae from pregnancies complicated by severe FGR and suspected fetal compromise (Denison et al. 2012). Further spectroscopy on the placenta of high-risk pregnancies, prior to overt FGR, will elucidate the predictive capabilities of these biomarkers.

Conclusion

Antenatal ultrasound examination of the fetus and placenta is likely to remain at the forefront of fetal screening and surveillance for the majority of women. Immerging 3D and 4D ultrasound may provide additional information in the future, although further research is required before their full implementation. While MRI is unlikely to ever become routine, it may aid in the management of pregnancies affected by extreme FGR and preterm birth. For these women, MRI determinations of placental structure and measures of function, including perfusion, oxygenation and metabolism, may facilitate improved stratification of risk.

REFERENCES

Alfirevic Z, Stampalija T, Gyte GM (2010) Fetal and umbilical Doppler ultrasound in normal pregnancy. *Cochrane Database Sys Rev (Online)*, p.CD001450. doi: http://dx.doi.org/10.1002/14651858.CD001450.pub3

Azpurua H, Funai EF, Coraluzzi LM et al. (2010) Determination of placental weight using two-dimensional sonography and volumetric mathematic modeling. *Am J Perinatol* 27: 151–155. doi: http://dx.doi.org/10.1055/s-0029-1234034

Baker PN, Johnson IR, Gowland PA et al. (1995) Measurement of fetal liver, brain and placental volumes with echo-planar magnetic resonance imaging. *Br J Obstet Gynecol* 102: 35–39. doi: http://dx.doi.org/10.1111/j.1471-0528.1995.tb09023.x

Baschat AA (2010) Ductus venosus Doppler for fetal surveillance in high-risk pregnancies. *Clin Obstet Gynecol* 53: 858–868. doi: http://dx.doi.org/10.1097/grf.0b013e3181fbb06d

Baschat AA, Gembruch U, Weiner CP, Harman CR (2003) Qualitative venous Doppler waveform analysis improves prediction of critical perinatal outcomes in preterm growth-restricted fetuses. *Ultrasound Obstet Gynecol* 22: 240–245. doi: http://dx.doi.org/10.1002/uog.149

Baschat AA, Gembruch U, Reiss I, Gortner L, Weiner CP, Harman CR (2000) Relationship between arterial and venous Doppler and perinatal outcome in fetal growth restriction. *Ultrasound Obstet Gynecol* 16: 407–413. doi: http://dx.doi.org/10.1046/j.1469-0705.2000.00284.x

Bozkurt N, Yigiter AB, Gokaslan H, Kavak ZN (2010) Correlations of fetal-maternal outcomes and first trimester 3-D placental volume/3-D power Doppler calculations. *Clin Exp Obstet Gynecol* 30(1): 26–28.

Cetin I, Alvino G (2009) Intrauterine growth restriction: Implications for placental metabolism and transport. A review. *Placenta* 30: 77–82. doi: http://dx.doi.org/10.1016/j.placenta.2008.12.006

Collins SL, Stevenson GN, Noble JA, Impey L (2012) Developmental changes in spiral artery blood flow in the human placenta observed with colour Doppler ultrasonography. *Placenta* 33(10): 782–787. doi: http://dx.doi.org/10.1016/j.placenta.2012.07.005

Costantini D, Walker M, Milligan N, Keating S, Kingdom J (2012) Pathologic basis of improving the screening utility of 2-dimensional placental morphology ultrasound. *Placenta* 33(10): 845–849. doi: http://dx.doi.org/10.1016/j.placenta.2012.07.010

Damodaram M, Story L, Eixarch E et al. (2010) Placental MRI in intrauterine fetal growth restriction. *Placenta* 31(6): 491–498. doi: http://dx.doi.org/10.1016/j.placenta.2010.03.001

Denison FC, Semple SI, Stock SJ, Walker J, Marshall I, Norman JE (2012) Novel use of proton magnetic resonance spectroscopy (1HMRS) to non-invasively assess placental metabolism. *PLoS ONE* 7(8): e42926. doi: http://dx.doi.org/10.1371/journal.pone.0042926

Derwig I, Lythgoe DJ, Barker GJ et al. (2013) Association of placental perfusion, as assessed by magnetic resonance imaging and uterine artery Doppler ultrasound, and its relationship to pregnancy outcome. *Placenta* 34(10): 885–891. doi: http://dx.doi.org/10.1016/j.placenta.2013.07.006

Derwig IE, Akolekar R, Zelaya FO, Gowland PA, Barker GJ, Nicolaides KH (2011) Association of placental volume measured by MRI and birth weight percentile. *Journal of Magnetic Resonance Imaging: JMRI* 34(5): 1125–1130. doi: http://dx.doi.org/10.1002/jmri.22794

Deurloo K, Spreeuwenberg M, Rekoert-Hollander M, van Vugt J (2007) Reproducibility of 3-dimensional sonographic measurements of fetal and placental volume at gestational ages of 11–18 weeks. *J Clin Ultrasound* 35: 125–132. doi: http://dx.doi.org/10.1002/jcu.20306

Fisteag-Kiprono L, Neiger R, Sonek JD, Croom CS, McKenna DS, Ventolini G (2006) Perinatal outcome associated with sonographically detected globular placenta. *J Reprod Med* 51: 563–566.

Francis ST, Duncan KR, Moore RJ, Baker PN, Johnson IR, Gowland PA (1998) Early reports non-invasive mapping of placental perfusion. *Lancet* 351: 1397–1399.

Gowland PA, Francis ST, Duncan KR et al. (1998) In vivo perfusion measurements in the human placenta using echo planar imaging at 0.5 T. *Magn Reson Med: Official Journal of the Society of Magnetic Resonance in Medicine / Society of Magnetic Resonance in Medicine* 40: 467–473. doi: http://dx.doi.org/10.1002/mrm.1910400318

Grannum PA, Berkowitz RL, Hobbins JC (1979) The ultrasonic changes in the maturing placenta and their relation to fetal pulmonic maturity. *Am J Obstet Gynecol* 133: 915–922.

Guiot C, Gaglioti P, Oberto M, Piccoli E, Rosato R, Todros T (2008) Is three-dimensional power Doppler ultrasound useful in the assessment of placental perfusion in normal and growth-restricted pregnancies? *Ultrasound Obstet Gynecol* 31(2): 171–176. doi: http://dx.doi.org/10.1002/uog.5212

Hafner E, Philipp T, Schuchter K, Dillinger-Paller B, Philipp K, Bauer P (1998) Second-trimester measurements of placental volume by three-dimensional ultrasound to predict small-for-gestational-age infants. *Ultrasound Obstet Gynecol* 12: 97–102. doi: http://dx.doi.org/10.1046/j.1469-0705.1998.12020097.x

Hata T, Tanaka H, Noguchi J, Hata K (2011) Three-dimensional ultrasound evaluation of the placenta. *Placenta* 32(2): 105–115. doi: http://dx.doi.org/10.1016/j.placenta.2010.11.001

Heazell AEP, Brown M, Dunn WB et al. (2008) Analysis of the metabolic footprint and tissue metabolome of placental villous explants cultured at different oxygen tensions reveals novel redox biomarkers. *Placenta* 29: 691–698. doi: http://dx.doi.org/10.1016/j.placenta.2008.05.002

Heinonen S, Taipale P, Saarikoski S (2001) Weights of placentae from small-for-gestational age infants revisited. *Placenta* 22: 399–404. doi: http://dx.doi.org/10.1053/plac.2001.0630

Hoddick WK, Mahony BS, Callen PW, Filly RA (1985) Placental thickness. *J Ultrasound Med: Official Journal of the American Institute of Ultrasound in Medicine* 4: 479–482.

Huen I, Morris DM, Wright C, Sibley CP, Naish JH, Johnstone ED (2014) Absence of PO2 change in fetal brain despite PO2 increase in placenta in response to maternal oxygen challenge. *BJOG* 121(13): 1588–1594. doi: http://dx.doi.org/10.1111/1471-0528.12804. Epub 2014 May 12.

Huen I, Morris DM, Wright C et al. (2013) R1 and R2* changes in the human placenta in response to maternal oxygen challenge. *Magn Reson Med: Official Journal of the Society of Magnetic Resonance in Medicine / Society of Magnetic Resonance in Medicine* 70(5): 1427–1433. doi: http://dx.doi.org/10.1002/mrm.24581

Jauniaux E, Watson A, Burton G (2001) Evaluation of respiratory gases and acid-base gradients in human fetal fluids and uteroplacental tissue between 7 and 16 weeks' gestation. *Am J Obstet Gynecol* 184: 998–1003. doi: http://dx.doi.org/10.1067/mob.2001.111935

Johnson P, Stojilkovic T, Sarkar P (2001) Middle cerebral artery Doppler in severe intrauterine growth restriction. *Ultrasound Obstet Gynecol* 17: 416–420. doi: http://dx.doi.org/10.1046/j.1469-0705.2001.00404.x

Kalache KD, Duckelmann AM (2012) Doppler in obstetrics. *Clin Obstet Gynecol* 55: 288–295.

Lee W, Kirk JS, Comstock CH, Romero R (2000) Vasa previa: Prenatal detection by three-dimensional ultrasonography. *Ultrasound Obstet Gynecol* 16(4): 384–387. doi: http://dx.doi.org/10.1046/j.1469-0705.2000.00188.x

Linduska N, Dekan S, Messerschmidt A et al. (2009) Placental pathologies in fetal MRI with pathohistological correlation. *Placenta* 30(6): 555–559. doi: http://dx.doi.org/10.1016/j.placenta.2009.03.010

Liu CC, Pretorius DH, Scioscia AL, Hull AD (2002) Sonographic prenatal diagnosis of marginal placental cord insertion: Clinical importance. *J Ultrasound Med* 21(6): 627–632.

March MI, Warsof SL, Chauhan SP (2012) Fetal biometry: Relevance in obstetrical practice. *Clin Obstet Gynecol* 55: 281–287. doi: http://dx.doi.org/10.1097/grf.0b013e3182446e9b

Marcos HB, Semelka RC, Worawattanakul S (1997) Normal placenta: Gadolinium-enhanced dynamic MR imaging. *Radiology* 205: 493–496. doi: http://dx.doi.org/10.1148/radiology.205.2.9356634

McKenna D, Tharmaratnam S, Mahsud S, Dornan J (2005) Ultrasonic evidence of placental calcification at 36 weeks' gestation: Maternal and fetal outcomes. *Acta Obstet Gynecol Scand* 84: 7–10. doi: http://dx.doi.org/10.1111/j.0001-6349.2005.00563.x

Meler E, Figueras F, Mula R et al. (2010) Prognostic role of uterine artery Doppler in patients with pre-eclampsia. *Fetal Diagn Ther* 27: 8–13.

Moore RJ, Strachan BK, Tyler DJ, Duncan KR, Baker PN, Worthington BS (2000) In utero perfusing fraction maps in normal and growth restricted pregnancy measured using IVIM echo-planar MRI. *Placenta* 21(7): 726–732.

Ong SS, Tyler DJ, Moore RJ et al. (2004) Functional magnetic resonance imaging (magnetization transfer) and stereological analysis of human placentae in normal pregnancy and in pre-eclampsia and intrauterine growth restriction. *Placenta* 25(5): 408–412.

Pretorius DH, Chau C, Poeltler DM, Mendoza A, Catanzarite VA, Hollenbach KA (1996) Placental cord insertion visualization with prenatal ultrasonography. *J Ultrasound Med: Official Journal of the American Institute of Ultrasound in Medicine* 15: 585–593.

Rizzo G, Capponi A, Pietrolucci M, Capece A, Arduini D (2009) First-trimester placental volume and vascularization measured by 3-Dimensional power Doppler sonography in pregnancies with low serum PAPPA levels. *J Ultrasound Med* 28(12): 1615–1622.

Rizzo G, Capponi A, Cavicchioni O, Vendola M, Arduini D (2008) First trimester uterine Doppler and three-dimensional ultrasound placental volume calculation in predicting pre-eclampsia. *Eur J Obstet Gynecol Reprod Biol* 138: 147–151. doi: http://dx.doi.org/10.1016/j.ejogrb.2007.08.015

Roberts N, Thilaganathan B (2007) The role of ultrasound in obstetrics. *Obstet Gynecol Reprod Med* 17: 79–85. doi: http://dx.doi.org/10.1016/j.ogrm.2006.12.014

Salafia CM, Charles AK, Maas EM (2006) Placenta and fetal growth restriction. *Clin Obstet Gynecol* 49: 236–256. doi: http://dx.doi.org/10.1097/00003081-200606000-00007

Sau A, Seed P, Langford K (2004) Intraobserver and interobserver variation in the sonographic grading of placental maturity. *Ultrasound Obstet Gynecol* 23: 374–377. doi: http://dx.doi.org/10.1002/uog.1004

Sciscione AC, Hayes EJ (2009) Uterine artery Doppler flow studies in obstetric practice. *Am J Obstet Gynecol* 201: 121–126. doi: http://dx.doi.org/10.1016/j.ajog.2009.03.027

Sibley CP, Turner MA, Cetin I et al. (2005) Placental phenotypes of intrauterine growth. *Pediatr Res* 58: 827–832. doi: http://dx.doi.org/10.1203/01.pdr.0000181381.82856.23

Simanaviciute D, Gudmundsson S (2006) Fetal middle cerebral to uterine artery pulsatility index ratios in normal and pre-eclamptic pregnancies. *Ultrasound Obstet Gynecol* 28: 794–801. doi: http://dx.doi.org/10.1002/uog.3805

Sohlberg S, Mulic-Lutvica A, Lindgren P, Ortiz-Nieto F, Wikström AK, Wikström J (2014) Placental perfusion in normal pregnancy and early and late preeclampsia: A magnetic resonance imaging study. *Placenta* 35(3): 202–206.

Sørensen A, Peters D, Fründ E, Lingman G, Christiansen O, Uldbjerg N (2013) Changes in human placental oxygenation during maternal hyperoxia estimated by blood oxygen level-dependent magnetic resonance imaging (BOLD MRI). *Ultrasound Obstet Gynecol* 42(3): 310–314. doi: http://dx.doi.org/10.1002/uog.12395

Story L, Damodaram MS, Allsop JM et al. (2011) Brain metabolism in fetal intrauterine growth restriction: A proton magnetic resonance spectroscopy study. *Am J Obstet Gynecol* 205: 483.e1–483.e8. doi: http://dx.doi.org/10.1016/j.ajog.2011.06.032

Story L, Damodaram MS, Allsop JM et al. (2011) Proton magnetic resonance spectroscopy in the fetus. *Eur J Obstet Gynecol Reprod Biol* 158(1): 3–8. doi: http://dx.doi.org/10.1016/j.ejogrb.2010.03.003

Toal M, Keating S, Machin G et al. (2008) Determinants of adverse perinatal outcome in high-risk women with abnormal uterine artery Doppler images. *Am J Obstet Gynecol* 198: 330.e1–330.e7. doi: http://dx.doi.org/10.1016/j.ajog.2007.09.031

Todros T, Sciarrone A, Piccoli E, Guiot C, Kaufmann P, Kingdom J (1999) Umbilical Doppler waveforms and placental villous angiogenesis in pregnancies complicated by fetal growth restriction. *Obstet Gynecol* 93: 499–503. doi: http://dx.doi.org/10.1016/s0029-7844(98)00440-2

Turan OM, Turan S, Gungor S et al. (2008) Progression of Doppler abnormalities in intrauterine growth restriction. *Ultrasound Obstet Gynecol* 32: 160–167. doi: http://dx.doi.org/10.1002/uog.5386

Welsh AW, Taylor MJO, Cosgrove D, Fisk NM (2001) Freehand three-dimensional Doppler demonstration of monochorionic vascular anastomoses in vivo: A preliminary report. *Ultrasound Obstet Gynecol* 18: 317–324. doi: http://dx.doi.org/10.1046/j.0960-7692.2001.00552.x

Wright C, Morris DM, Baker PN et al. (2011) Magnetic resonance imaging relaxation time measurements of the placenta at 1.5T. *Placenta* 32(12): 1010–1015. doi: http://dx.doi.org/10.1016/j.placenta.2011.07.008

Yampolsky M, Salafia CM, Shlakhter O et al. (2009) Centrality of the umbilical cord insertion in a human placenta influences the placental efficiency. *Placenta* 30: 1058–1064.

9
CEREBRAL FUNCTION AND FETAL GROWTH RESTRICTION

Irene Cetin and Valentina Brusati

As noted in Chapter 2, fetal growth restriction (FGR) due to placental insufficiency has been correlated to a specific placental phenotype based on the evidence that defective fetal nutrition is related to a progressive deterioration in placental function, that is, a decrease in transplacental transfer of oxygen and nutrients (Sibley et al. 2005). The resulting fetal hypoxaemia is a major stimulus in the reduction in fetal growth, as an attempt to reduce metabolic demands by the growing fetus. This impaired placental function will alter the development of the fetal vasculature, organs or signalling pathways in ways that predispose the fetus to later developmental disease (Barker et al. 1990). This chapter will focus on available data and hypotheses explaining how FGR can attenuate and perturb normal cerebral development.

Critical stages of fetal brain development
Cerebral development is a complex and long-lasting process with continuous neurobiological changes occurring throughout pre- and postnatal life. These periods of specific neurodevelopmental events result in windows of vulnerability for adverse influence. Before trying to shed light on mechanisms which disrupt fetal brain development in the growth restricted fetus, we will briefly review events, in sequence, which take place during ontogeny of the human nervous system.

In the first half of human pregnancy, neuronal proliferation and migration are especially vigorous. The majority of neurons are generated during the first 20 weeks' gestation, except for granule cells of the olfactory bulb, cerebellum and hippocampus, which continue genesis after birth. Once neurons have been generated, they move from their place of origin to their final destination. In the human cerebral cortex, migration takes place from the early phases of brain development, peaks between the third and fifth month of pregnancy and stops around 30 weeks' post-menstrual age (PMA). During migration, neurons start to differentiate, but a major part of axon and dendrite sprouting occurs when the cells have reached their final positions (de Graaf-Peters and Hadders-Algra 2006).

The second half of gestation is characterized by major glial cell proliferation, programmed cell death and existence of the transient structure called the 'subplate'. The subplate is functionally important as a temporary goal of afferent fibres, playing a role in the guidance of some corticofugal pathways and contributing to the early and transient cortical neuronal circuits involved in the generation of fetal behaviour. The subplate emerges during early fetal life, is thickest around 29 weeks' PMA, regresses after 31 weeks' PMA and then finally disappears.

During the last trimester and first postnatal year, axon and dendrite sprouting and synapse formation bloom. Corticospinal axons reach the lower cervical spinal cord by 26 weeks' PMA and then progressively and extensively innervate the spinal neurons, including the motor neurons. Dendritic development and synaptic formation accelerate, resulting in a sixfold increase in synaptic density by 28 weeks' PMA.

Although myelination starts early during gestation (12–14 weeks, of PMA), its synthesis increases in the latter half of pregnancy and first postnatal year. Myelin is a fatty insulating sheath, which surrounds axons and promotes rapid and efficient impulse conductions. Myelin is produced by glial cells, the oligodendrocytes. Progenitors of these cells in the periventricular white matter are abundantly present till 27 weeks' PMA; thereafter, they mature into myelin producing cells. It is noteworthy that in humans, the late precursor cells (pre-oligodendrocytes) and immature oligodendrocytes that predominate in the developing periventricular white matter during the period of highest risk of damage (23–32 weeks of postconceptional age) are particularly susceptible to hypoxic-ischaemic injury (de Graaf-Peters and Hadders-Algra 2006, Rees et al. 2011).

During normal brain development, regressive phenomena are also active. Programmed cell death, commonly referred to as 'apoptosis' and axon retraction are the two prominent regressive processes to ensure the formation and plasticity of appropriate neuronal networks (de Graaf-Peters and Hadders-Algra 2006). As well as these physical changes, neurotransmitters and neuromodulary substances play an important regulatory role in developing the nervous system, affecting neural migration, differentiation and especially contributing to orchestrating and shaping synaptic circuitry. The major neurotransmitters (catecholamines, acetylcholine, glutamate and gamma-aminobutyric acid [GABA]) are present from a very early age. With glutamate receptors abundant in early life, the immature brain is particularly vulnerable to excitotoxic injury.

In this context, it is clear that the clinical consequences of adverse conditions during prenatal life depend both on the nature and the severity of the insult and also on the timing of specific neurodevelopmental events. A well-known clinical example of this age-dependent effect is the difference in the impact of perinatal asphyxia or hypoxic-ischaemic disease in preterm and term infants. Lesions due to perinatal asphyxia in preterm infants are usually localised in the periventricular regions, whereas in term infants, the cortical areas, thalamus, basal ganglia and brainstem show specific vulnerability (de Graaf-Peters and Hadders-Algra 2006).

In summary, brain development is highly active during the second half of pregnancy, when fetal growth restriction may become clinically evident. This period includes the initiation of myelination, axonal and dendritic growth, synaptogenesis and proliferation of microglia and astrocytes.

Neurostructural and cerebral vascular modifications in growth restriction
ANATOMY AND ANIMAL MODELS

The relevance of the brain in fetal-neonatal physiology is evident from its large size in the newborn infant. Data on brain/body weight ratios were originally obtained by pathologists from autopsies on stillborn and dead newborn infants. These data showed that the brain/ total body weight ratio declines slowly between 20 and 30 weeks' gestation and remains virtually constant around 0.13 from 30 weeks to term. Figure 9.1 shows the percentage brain weights of newborn infants and adults in several species (Cross 1979). It is noteworthy that the ratio between brain and body weight is significantly higher in newborn infants than in adults in all species and that this phenomenon is particularly evident in humans with a ratio about six times higher than the adult (0.13 vs. 0.02). Furthermore, in the newborn infant the brain is more than twice the weight of the liver, while in adult life the liver is the heavier and ratio nearer to 1 (Pardi and Cetin 2006).

The increased growth of the fetal brain in second half gestation is paralleled by the increased deposition of essential fatty acids (Clandinin et al. 1980). In FGR pregnancies, differences in the relative amounts of fetal and maternal plasma fatty acids have been observed (Cetin et al. 2002). Since fatty acids are utilised for neural tissue synthesis, these differences might have a role in determining the biochemical environment leading to the neural and vascular complications associated with FGR.

Human autopsy studies on FGR infants have shown that although the brain is relatively spared compared with other organs, brain weights are reduced by 15–25% compared with controls, whereas liver, lungs and thymus are more profoundly affected, with weight reductions of more than 50% (Pardi and Cetin 2006).

Brain damage due to FGR has been studied in animal models during the second half of gestation. The brain, although relatively spared in relation to other organs, was found to

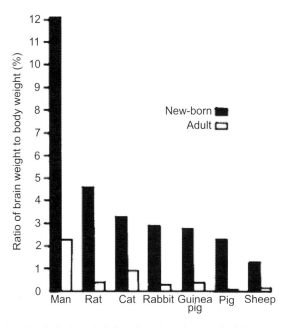

Fig. 9.1. The ratio of brain:body weight in selected newborn and adult mammals. Reproduced from *J Physiol* 294: 1–21, with permission from John Wiley and Sons Ltd.

be reduced in weight in induced FGR sheep and guinea pig fetuses. No overt white matter damage was detected, although axonal myelination was delayed in the central nervous system (CNS) (Rees et al. 2011). Chronic intrauterine insults seem to compromise the growth of neural processes and synapses throughout the fetal sheep and guinea pig brain examined at term. Neurons generally survive chronic, mild intrauterine compromise, although some populations are affected; reduced cell numbers could relate to a direct effect of hypoxia on neurogenesis or alternatively to the death of post-mitotic cells. The reduction in cortical growth and decrease in cell number in the future cortex have also been found in severely affected human FGR infants, studied at autopsy by optical fractionators (Samuelsen et al. 2007).

The guinea pig model of chronic placental insufficiency has contributed also to the neurodevelopmental hypothesis of schizophrenia. Ventriculomegaly is one of the most consistent findings in the brains of patients with schizophrenia and studies on guinea pig models of FGR demonstrated that such alterations can originate from chronic insults in utero. It was suggested that the enlargement of the lateral ventricles observed in guinea pig FGR fetuses most likely resulted from reduced growth of neural processes and reduced neuronal numbers in some brain regions (Rees and Inder 2005). For more information on this topic, see Chapter 10.

METABOLIC MEASURES OF CEREBRAL IMPAIRMENT

The brain is not only a relatively 'large' organ, but also a 'demanding' one. In fact, in adults at rest the brain consumes up to 18% of total oxygen consumption, despite its weight representing only 2% of total body weight. In physiological conditions, the CNS has a relatively high requirement for oxygen and glucose mostly metabolised by oxidative phosphorylation. The brain is a metabolically demanding organ even at birth and its expenses are directed to immediate use, as well as its future potential (Sanders et al. 2010).

As discussed so far, the aetiology of brain damage due to FGR is likely to be multifactorial. However, reduced oxygen delivery to the developing brain and its downstream effects play a major role. Changes in energy metabolism associated with adaptations to chronic hypoxia and hypoglycaemia in utero are important determinants of susceptibility to perinatal hypoxic brain injury in FGR neonates. In the fetal brain, energy is primarily derived from metabolism of glucose via the Krebs cycle and oxidative phosphorylation in the mitochondria (36 mol ATP/mol glucose) and to a lesser extent by glycolysis in the cytosol (2 mol ATP/mol glucose). Inhibition of oxidative phosphorylation during acute hypoxia decreases energy generation in the brain resulting in energy deficiency, cellular injury and cell death (Moxon-Lester et al. 2007, Rees et al. 2011).

As mentioned above, FGR is a condition that can be associated with chronic fetal hypoxia and acidaemia (Pardi et al. 1993, Cetin and Alvino 2009). Fetal acidemia rather than hypoxaemia carries the greater risk for irreversible developmental delay and the likelihood of acidemia increases with clinical signs of fetal deterioration. Plasma lactic acid concentration is a well-known marker of acidemia and low oxygen delivery to peripheral tissues. In fact, lactate is the end product of anaerobic glycolysis and its concentration increases when the normal aerobic mechanism fails. Plasma lactic acid concentration is higher in FGR fetuses with altered umbilical arterial Doppler velocimetry and abnormal fetal heart rate (Marconi et al. 1990, Pardi et al. 1993). However, little is known about intrauterine changes in cerebral metabolism in these conditions.

As outlined in Chapter 8, recent years have seen the emergence of a new imaging modality with which to investigate fetal brain metabolism (Brighina et al. 2009), proton magnetic resonance spectroscopy (^{1}H-MRS). This non-invasive technique identifies *in vivo* several metabolites of biological importance, including lactate. While at normal concentrations lactate is hardly visible in the brain by MRS, under anaerobic conditions its concentration increases and signal appears (van der Graaf 2010). Indeed, elevated levels of lactate detected by ^{1}H-MRS in the brain of asphyxiated neonates have been found to be predictive of neurodevelopmental delay (Barkovich et al. 1999, Roelants-van Rijn et al. 2004a).

The metabolic profile of the fetal brain has also been described in utero by ^{1}H-MRS, during the second and third trimesters of uncomplicated pregnancies (Girard et al. 2006a, Girard et al. 2006b). Again, such studies have failed to detect lactate in the normal fetal brain, leading to several authors suggesting that the evidence of cerebral lactate could represent an indicator of altered fetal cerebral metabolism in pathological conditions (Roelants-van Rijn et al. 2004b, Wolfberg et al. 2007, Azpurua et al. 2008). During experimental-induced fetal hypoxia in pregnant sheep, MRS has indeed shown large increases in fetal brain lactate levels (van Cappellen et al. 1999). Moreover, in the experimental study on newborn piglets, increased brain lactate in animals subjected to mild hypoxia was directly associated with intrauterine growth restriction (Moxon-Lester et al. 2007).

Recently, three studies have evaluated fetal brain metabolism by MRS in human FGR (Charles-Edwards et al. 2010, Cetin et al. 2011, Story et al. 2011). The first report found the presence of lactate in all four cases regardless of FGR severity (Charles-Edwards et al. 2010). In another series of five FGR fetuses, lactate peak was detected only in the most severely compromised and lactacidemic (Cetin et al. 2011) (Fig. 9.2). These two studies support the concept of lactate as a possible marker of altered cerebral metabolism in severe FGR fetuses, although its clinical relevance on long-term outcome still requires evaluation. In the last study, lactate was identified in some FGR but also in some appropriately grown fetuses (5 out of 41 and 3 out of 28 fetuses respectively). Nevertheless, reduced ratios between N-acetylaspartate (NAA, a neuronal marker) and choline (a marker of myelination and cell membrane synthesis) were defined, suggesting that brain metabolism was altered in the growth restricted fetuses (Story et al. 2011). This decrease in NAA in FGR fetuses may reflect impaired neuronal mitochondrial function and metabolism. Conversely, a recent study conducted by MRS on 28 growth-restricted fetuses compared with 48 appropriately grown comparison fetuses showed that FGR is not associated with differences in brain myo-inositol ratio (Story et al. 2013).

Functional evaluation of brain integrity

Today, the best available tool for the evaluation of neurological integrity in utero is still represented by fetal heart rate (FHR) analysis. Since FHR patterns are regulated by the autonomic nervous system, at a higher cortical level of the CNS, FHR variability must indeed be considered as an indicator of neurological rather than cardiac function in the fetus (Pardi and Cetin 2006).

Alterations in FHR patterns in human FGR fetuses are characterised by a reduction in FHR variability, a reduction in the number of FHR accelerations and a lack of an inverse relationship between baseline FHR and the amplitude of FHR accelerations when compared with normally grown fetuses. This abnormal FHR pattern has been described as 'immature', because of its similarity to normal FHR patterns seen before 30 weeks' gestation (Gagnon 2003). In fetal sheep with induced severe placental insufficiency, the normal maturational increase in FHR variability occurring with advancing gestation is abolished all together, with a 50% reduction in the number of accelerations (Gagnon 2003). Moreover, a mean variability below 1 beat/min strongly implies the disappearance of heart rate control and can be viewed as a sign of CNS lesions.

Experimental studies of electrocortical activity in similar ovine models of placental insufficiency have provided further evidence of abnormal neurodevelopment in response to chronic hypoxaemia. Normal electrocorticography (ECoG) recordings reveal alternating

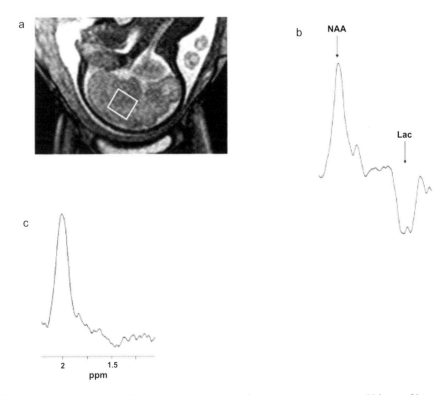

Fig. 9.2. Fetal brain lactate detection by proton magnetic resonance spectroscopy. Volume of interest (white box) shown in T2-weighted MR sagittal image (a). Proton spectra represented on the left. (b) Severe FGR with lactate clearly detectable. (c) Less severe FGR of similar gestational age. Lac, lactate; NAA, N-acetylaspartate Reprinted from: Lactate detection in the human fetal brain of intrauterine growth restricted (IUGR) fetuses: A 1-H magnetic resonance spectroscopy study, *Am J Obstet Gynecol* 205: 350.e1–350.e7, with permission from Elsevier.

periods of low-voltage/high-frequency (LV/HF) electrocortical activity, indicative of behavioural states related to cortical neuronal activity. In these ovine models, ECoG activity is significantly altered in response to chronic induced hypoxia (Frasch et al. 2011).

Short-term cerebral impairment

In FGR fetuses, the risk of complications in postnatal life reflects both the liabilities of intrauterine compromise and the penalties of preterm birth, with the combination worse than those of preterm birth alone. In a large prospective international multicentre study, evaluating growth-restricted fetuses with multi-vessel Doppler, the impact of fetal cardiovascular and perinatal variables on critical neonatal outcomes has been quantified (Baschat et al. 2007). In this study, severe intraventricular haemorrhage (IVH) was the second most frequent neonatal complication after bronchopulmonary dysplasia, affecting around 15% of the FGR population. Intraventricular haemorrhage was significantly related to gestational age, with the highest rates between 25 and 28 weeks' gestation.

Whether FGR is a condition at increased risk of IVH and white matter lesions has not been clarified. However, early studies suggested that small for gestational age is associated with a reduced incidence of IVH and periventricular leukomalacia (PVL) (Procianoy et al. 1980, Amato et al 1993). Recent studies have failed to confirm this connection (Larroque et al. 2003, Garite et al. 2004, Ramenghi et al. 2011) and one has even shown an increased incidence of IVH in FGR newborn infants (Zaw et al. 2003).

In another study, the prevalence of transient periventricular echodensities (TPE), PVL and haemorrhagic brain lesions, assessed by serial neonatal brain ultrasound in a group of preterm FGR neonates, was compared with preterm appropriate for gestational age (AGA) infants matched for gestational age at delivery (Padilla-Gomes 2007). FGR neonates had a significantly increased prevalence of TPE and PVL. Although the impact of TPE was milder than that of PVL, TPE was associated with abnormal motor and cognitive neurodevelopment, suggestive of white matter damage (Padilla-Gomes 2007).

Long-term cerebral impairment

The long-term neurological and cognitive development of FGR infants has been extensively studied. Several reports have supported the notion that FGR is associated with a higher incidence of perinatal complications and is associated with specific long-term neurodevelopmental sequels. Nevertheless, it has been difficult to tease out the relative effects of severity of growth restriction from those of preterm birth (Kok et al. 2007, Leitner et al. 2000, Leitner et al. 2007). Long-term morbidity ranges from behavioural problems and minor developmental delay to spastic cerebral palsy. Such a large spectrum of neurological impairments could have several explanations, but perhaps again reflects the dynamism of the fetal brain and its disparate response depending on onset, duration and intensity of the injury.

As discussed, during the second half of gestation profound changes in brain organization take place, involving critical neural connections and myelination of important neural tracts (de Graaf-Peters et al. 2006). It is not known how susceptibility of the brain changes with maturation, but it is plausible that even mild degrees of hypoxia could induce permanent epigenetic changes as part of adaptation of the developing brain to a hypoxic and undernourished environment (Cruz-Martinez et al. 2009). Different responses might have different neurological manifestations. Nevertheless, diverse neurodevelopmental outcomes could be determined by biological factors modulated by the subsequent psychosocial environment.

Recent long-term postnatal studies have demonstrated that FGR is specifically associated with significant neurodevelopmental deficits that cannot be attributed to preterm birth alone. Different reports from various cohorts around the world suggest that children born with FGR tend to have a general mild deficit in IQ persisting through their adult life. Performance is usually within the normal range for the child's age, but lower than that attained by well-matched controls, whose weight at birth has been adequately adjusted for gestational age.

Whether the deficit in IQ arises from a general intellectual deficit or from specific neuropsychological shortfalls has yet to be clarified. The former hypothesis may be accounted for by a general effect of growth restriction on brain maturation as a whole, while the latter is based on the notion that certain brain systems are more susceptible to FGR, relative to others (Geva et al. 2012). A long-term prospective study conducted on a large cohort of children born with FGR yielded a neuropsychological profile (Geva et al. 2006). In particular, FGR-born children scored lower than controls in domains that probe associative areas and the higher order association cortex. Specific cognitive neuropsychological functions affected by FGR are as follows: sensory motor, language, visuospatial, memory, attention, executive functions and learning functions and socio-emotional functioning. This report also suggested that neuropsychological dysfunction could be explained by increased prevalence of white matter injury.

Somatic catch-up growth also has implications on specific neuropsychological functions in addition to IQ. Catch-up growth has a remedial effect on most of the academic domains, in particular on language-based skills and on arithmetic skills and complete catch-up is more effective than a selected one. That is, children born with FGR whose head circumference, weight and height are greater than the 10th centile by 3 years of age tend to have significantly higher general knowledge attainment and arithmetic skills relative to children born with FGR who exhibit catch-up growth in only one of these dimensions or that do not exhibit catch-up growth at all by the first 3 years of age (Geva et al. 2012).

Conclusions

FGR is a condition associated with considerable perinatal risk and its influence can extend over a lifetime. The developmental origins of health and disease hypothesis opens fundamental new perspectives on preventing late-onset disease and disorders. The brain is particularly vulnerable to hypoxic damage resulting in short- and long-term impairments. In order to provide timely therapeutic intervention for the fetus or infant at risk of brain damage, we need to be able to detect when an insult has occurred by identifying reliable markers of brain damage. Basic questions that still need to be addressed are (1) How should we decide timing of delivery to improve neurological outcome? and (2) Can we protect the fetal brain from hypoxic insults?

At present we still lack specific clinical tools to accurately predict when the fetus enters the failure phase and needs to be delivered and/or should receive neuroprotective treatment. Defining the natural history of brain injury is crucial if we are to develop rational neuroprotective strategies to reduce the burden of altered brain growth and poor functional and behavioural outcomes. An advantage of the use of preconditioning strategies is to potentiate endogenous neuroprotective mechanisms before the insult occurs. Neuroprotective preconditioning, which was first described by Murry et al. (1986) in the ischaemic myocardium, is a process by which a tissue is rendered more tolerant to a subsequent lethal insult, such as ischaemia. As the mechanisms of hypoxic preconditioning are further unravelled, it is anticipated that pharmacological agents can be developed to activate these cellular defence mechanisms. Priorities for future research must include going beyond diagnosis of FGR, to improving placental function in utero. As a final goal, success in these endeavours would promote intrauterine growth, prolong gestation and reduce the risks of hypoxia.

REFERENCES

Amato M, Konrad D, Huppi P, Donati F (1993) Impact of prematurity and intrauterine growth retardation on neonatal hemorrhagic and ischemic brain damage. *Eur Neurol* 33: 299–303. doi: http://dx.doi.org/10.1159/000116958.

Azpurua H, Alvarado A, Mayobre F, Salom T, Copel J, Guevara-Zuloaga F (2008) Metabolic assessment of the brain using proton magnetic resonance spectroscopy in a growth-restricted human fetus: Case report. *Am J Perinatol* 25: 305–309. doi: http://dx.doi.org/10.1055/s-2008-1076603.

Barker DJ (1990) The fetal and infant origins of adult disease. *BMJ* 301: 1111. doi: http://dx.doi.org/10.1136/bmj.301.6761.1111.

Barkovich AJ, Barnski K, Vigneron D et al. (1999) Proton MR spectroscopy for the evaluation of brain injury in asphyxiated term neonates. *AJNR Am J Neuroradiol* 20: 1399–1405.

Baschat AA, Cosmi E, Bilardo CM et al. (2007) Predictors of neonatal outcome in early-onset placental dysfunction. *Obstet Gynecol* 109: 253–261. doi: http://dx.doi.org/10.1097/01.aog.0000253215.79121.75.

Brighina E, Bresolin N, Pardi G, Rango M (2009) Human fetal brain chemistry as detected by proton magnetic resonance spectroscopy. *Pediat Neurol* 40: 327–341. doi: http://dx.doi.org/10.1016/j.pediatrneurol.2008.11.001.

Cetin I, Alvino G (2009) Intrauterine growth restriction: Implications for placental metabolism and transport. A review. *Placenta* 30: 77–82. doi: http://dx.doi.org/10.1016/j.placenta.2008.12.006.

Cetin I, Barberis B, Brusati V et al. (2011) Lactate detection in the human fetal brain of intrauterine growth restricted (IUGR) fetuses: A 1-H magnetic resonance spectroscopy study. *Am J Obstet Gynecol* 205: 350.e1–350.e7. doi: http://dx.doi.org/10.1016/j.ajog.2011.06.020.

Cetin I, Giovannini N, Alvino G et al. (2002) Intrauterine growth restriction is associated with changes in polyunsaturated fatty acid fetal-maternal relationships. *Pediatr Res* 52: 750–755. doi: http://dx.doi.org/10.1203/00006450-200211000-00023.

Charles-Edwards GD, Jan W, To M, Maxwell D, Keevil SF, Robinson R (2010) Non-invasive detection and quantification of human foetal brain lactate in utero by magnetic resonance spectroscopy. *Prenat Diagn* 30: 260–266. doi: http://dx.doi.org/10.1002/pd.2463.

Clandinin MT, Chappell JE, Leong S, Heim T, Swyer PR, Chance GW (1980) Intrauterine fatty acid accretion rates in human brain: Implications for fatty acid requirements. *Early Hum Dev* 4: 121–129. doi: http://dx.doi.org/10.1016/0378-3782(80)90015-8.

Cross K W (1979) La chaleur animale and the infant brain. *J Physiol* 294: 1–21. doi: http://dx.doi.org/10.1113/jphysiol.1979.sp012911.

Cruz-Martinez R, Figueras F, Oros D et al. (2009) Cerebral blood perfusion and neurobehavioral performance in full-term small-for-gestational-age fetuses. *Am J Obstet Gynecol* 201: 474.e1–474.e7. doi: http://dx.doi.org/10.1016/j.ajog.2009.05.028.

de Graaf-Peters VB, Hadders-Algra M (2006) Ontogeny of the human central nervous system: What is happening when? *Early Hum Dev* 82: 257–266. doi: http://dx.doi.org/10.1016/j.earlhumdev.2005.10.013.

Frasch MG, Keen AE, Gagnon R, Ross MG, Richardson BS (2011) Monitoring fetal electrocortical activity during labour for predicting worsening acidemia: A prospective study in the ovine fetus near term. *PLoS ONE* 6: e22100. doi: http://dx.doi.org/10.1371/journal.pone.0022100.

Gagnon R (2003) Placental insufficiency and its consequences. *Eur J Obstet Gynecol Reprod Biol* 110: S99–S107. doi: http://dx.doi.org/10.1016/s0301-2115(03)00179-9.

Garite TJ, Clark R, Thorp JA (2004) Intrauterine growth restriction increases morbidity and mortality among premature neonates. *Am J Obstet Gynecol* 191: 481–487. doi: http://dx.doi.org/10.1016/j.ajog.2004.01.036.

Geva R, Eshel R, Leitner Y, Valevski AF, Harel S (2006) Neuropsychological outcome of children with intrauterine growth restriction: A 9-year prospective study. *Pediatrics* 118: 91–100. doi: http://dx.doi.org/10.1542/peds.2005-2343.

Geva R, Leitner Y, Harel S (2012) Children born with intrauterine growth restriction: Neurodevelopmental outcome. In: Preedy VR, editor. *Handbook of Growth and Growth Monitoring in Health and Disease,* 193–208. New York: Springer.

Girard N, Fogliarini C, Viola A et al. (2006a) MRS of normal and impaired fetal brain development. *Europ J Radiol* 57: 217–225. doi: http://dx.doi.org/10.1016/j.ejrad.2005.11.021.

Girard N, Gouny SC, Viola A et al. (2006b) Assessment of normal fetal brain maturation in utero by proton magnetic resonance spectroscopy. *Magn Reson Med* 56: 768–775. doi: http://dx.doi.org/10.1002/mrm.21017.

Kok JH, Prick L, Merckel E, Everhard Y, Verkerk GJ, Scherjon SA (2007) Visual function at 11 years of age in preterm-born children with and without fetal brain sparing. *Pediatrics* 119: e1342–e1350. doi: http://dx.doi.org/10.1542/peds.2005-2857.

Larroque B, Marret S, Ancel PY et al. EPIPAGE Study Group (2003) White matter damage and intraventricular hemorrhage in very preterm infants: The EPIPAGE Study. *J Pediatr* 143: 477–483. doi: http://dx.doi.org/10.1067/s0022-3476(03)00417-7.

Leitner Y, Fattal-Valevski A, Geva R et al. (2000) Six-year follow-up of children with intrauterine growth retardation: Long-term, prospective study. *J Child Neurol* 15: 781–786. doi: http://dx.doi.org/10.1177/088307380001501202.

Leitner Y, Fattal-Valevski A, Geva R et al. (2007) Neurodevelopmental outcome of children with intrauterine growth retardation: A longitudinal, 10-year prospective study. *J Child Neurol* 22: 580–587. doi: http://dx.doi.org/10.1177/0883073807302605.

Marconi AM, Cetin I, Ferrazzi E, Ferrari MM, Pardi G, Battaglia FC (1990) Lactate metabolism in normal and growth-retarded human fetuses. *Pediatr Res* 28: 652–656. doi: http://dx.doi.org/10.1203/00006450-199012000-00022.

Moxon-Lester L, Sinclair K, Burke C, Cowin GJ, Rose SE, Colditz P (2007) Increased cerebral lactate during hypoxia may be neuroprotective in newborn piglets with intrauterine growth restriction. *Brain Res* 1179: 79–88. doi: http://dx.doi.org/10.1016/j.brainres.2007.08.037.

Murry CE, Jennings RB, Reimer KA (1986) Preconditioning with ischemia: A delay of lethal cell injury in ischemic myocardium. *Circulation* 74: 1124–1136. doi: http://dx.doi.org/10.1161/01.cir.74.5.1124.

Padilla-Gomes NF, Enríquez G, Acosta-Rojas R, Perapoch J, Hernandez-Andrade E, Gratacos E (2007) Prevalence of neonatal ultrasound brain lesions in premature infants with and without intrauterine growth restriction. *Acta Paediatr* 96: 1582–1587. doi: http://dx.doi.org/10.1111/j.1651-2227.2007.00496.x.

Pardi G, Cetin I (2006) Human fetal growth and organ development: Fifty years of discoveries. *Am J Obstet Gynecol* 194: 1088–1099. doi: http://dx.doi.org/10.1016/j.ajog.2005.12.056.

Pardi G, Cetin I, Marconi AM et al. (1993) Diagnostic value of blood sampling in fetuses with growth retardation. *N Engl J Med* 328: 692–696. doi: http://dx.doi.org/10.1056/nejm199303113281004.

Procianoy RS, Garcia-Prats JA, Adams JM, Silvers A, Rudolph AJ (1980) Hyaline membrane disease and intraventricular haemorrhage in small for gestational age infants. *Arch Dis Child* 55: 502–505. doi: http://dx.doi.org/10.1136/adc.55.7.502.

Ramenghi LA, Martinelli A, De Carli A et al. (2011) Cerebral maturation in IUGR and appropriate for gestational age preterm babies. *Reprod Sci* 18: 469–475. doi: http://dx.doi.org/10.1177/1933719110388847.

Rees S, Harding R, Walker D (2011) The biological basis of injury and neuroprotection in the fetal and neonatal brain. *Int J Dev Neurosci* 29: 551–563. doi: http://dx.doi.org/10.1016/j.ijdevneu.2011.04.004.

Rees S, Inder T (2005) Fetal and neonatal origins of altered brain development. *Early Hum Dev* 81: 753–761. doi: http://dx.doi.org/10.1016/j.earlhumdev.2005.07.004.

Roelants-van Rijn A, van der Grond J, Stigter R, de Vries LS, Groenendaal F (2004a) Cerebral structure and metabolism and long-term outcome in small-for-gestational-age preterm neonates. *Pediatr Res* 56: 285–290. doi: http://dx.doi.org/10.1203/01.pdr.0000132751.09067.3f.

Roelants-van Rijn AM, Groenendaal F, Stoutenbeek P, van der Grond J (2004b) Lactate in the foetal brain: Detection and implications. *Acta Paediatr* 93: 937–940. doi: http://dx.doi.org/10.1111/j.1651-2227.2004. tb02692.x.

Samuelsen GB, Pakkenberg B, Bogdanovi N et al. (2007) Severe cell reduction in the future brain cortex in human growth restricted fetuses and infants. *Am J Obstet Gynecol* 197: 56.e1–56.e7. doi: http://dx.doi.org/10.1016/j.ajog.2007.02.011.

Sanders RD, Manning HJ, Robertson NJ et al. (2010) Preconditioning and postinsult therapies for perinatal hypoxic-ischemic injury at term. *Anesthesiology* 113: 233–249. doi: http://dx.doi.org/10.1097/ aln.0b013e3181dc1b84.

Sibley CP, Turner MA, Cetin I et al. (2005) Placental phenotypes of intrauterine growth. *Pediatr Res* 58: 827–832. doi: http://dx.doi.org/10.1203/01.pdr.0000181381.82856.23.

Story L, Damodaram MS, Allsop JM et al. (2011) Brain metabolism in fetal intrauterine growth restriction: A proton magnetic resonance spectroscopy study. *Am J Obstet Gynecol* 205: 483.e1–483.e8. doi: http://dx.doi.org/10.1016/j.ajog.2011.06.032.

Story L, Damodaram MS, Supramaniam V et al. (2013) Myo-inositol metabolism in appropriately grown and growth-restricted fetuses: A proton magnetic resonance spectroscopy study. *Eur J Obstet Gynecol Reprod Biol* 170(1): 77–81. doi: http://dx.doi.org/10.1016/j.ejogrb.2013.05.006.

Van Cappellen AM, Heerschap A, Nijhuis JG, Oeseburg B, Jongsma HW (1999) Hypoxia, the subsequent systemic metabolic acidosis, and their relationship with cerebral metabolite concentration: An in vivo study in fetal lambs with proton magnetic resonance spectroscopy. *Am J Obstet Gynecol* 181: 1537–1545. doi: http://dx.doi.org/10.1016/s0002-9378(99)70401-1.

Van der Graaf M (2010) In vivo magnetic resonance spectroscopy: Basic methodology and clinical applications. *Eur Biophys J* 39: 527–540. doi: http://dx.doi.org/10.1007/s00249-009-0517-y.

Wolfberg AJ, Robinson JN, Mulkern R, Rybicki F, Du Plessis AJ (2007) Identification of fetal cerebral lactate using magnetic resonance spectroscopy. *Am J Obstet Gynecol* 196: e9–e11. doi: http://dx.doi.org/10.1016/j.ajog.2006.09.036.

Zaw W, Gagnon R, Silva O (2003) The risks of adverse neonatal outcome among preterm small for gestational age infants according to neonatal versus fetal growth standards. *Pediatrics* 111: 1273–1277. doi: http://dx.doi.org/10.1542/peds.111.6.1273.

10
PLACENTAL PROGRAMMING AND MENTAL ILLNESS: FETAL GROWTH AND SCHIZOPHRENIA

Kathryn Abel and Matthew Allin

Schizophrenia is a disabling, usually chronic condition with a lifetime prevalence of around 1%. It is characterised by heterogeneous symptoms including delusions, hallucinations and cognitive impairments and 'negative' symptoms such as emotional blunting and lack of motivation. The onset of symptoms is most common between 18 and 30 years, although it may begin in later life and, rarely, in childhood. Mean age at onset is typically about 5 years younger in males, although the modal age at onset is very similar between the sexes, at around 21 years of age.

Schizophrenia is conceptualised as a disorder of neurodevelopment. There is ample evidence that schizophrenia is associated with subtle abnormalities of brain structure and function. Twin studies originally suggested that schizophrenia is highly heritable (perhaps approaching 80%) (Cardno et al. 1999), but despite this it has proved difficult to isolate 'candidate genes' consistently across or within populations. More recently, genome-wide association studies and copy number variation studies suggest a role for both common and rare large copy number variations in schizophrenia, most notably those associated with genetic markers in the major histocompatibility complex (6p22.1), that is, NOTCH4 and histone protein loci (Tiwari et al. 2010) and deletions of NRXN1 which encode the synaptic scaffolding protein neurexin 1 (Doherty et al. 2012). In reality, the aetiology of schizophrenia requires interactions of these susceptibility genes, either singly or in combination, with a myriad of additional environment factors.

Aetiological mechanisms in schizophrenia must take account of the effects of 'social environment' widely evidenced by epidemiological findings. Risk factors include winter–spring season of birth, urban birth, birth complications, city living, migration, prenatal exposure to famine and maternal pregnancy-related infections. Abnormalities of fetal growth (in particular extremes of deviant growth) are consistently related to risk of neurodevelopmental disorder and schizophrenia with male early-onset illness. This chapter focuses on these social environmental risk factors for schizophrenia and, in particular, considers the effects associated with abnormalities of fetal growth.

Schizophrenia as a disorder of neurodevelopment
The concept of schizophrenia as a condition with origins in early brain development goes back to the late nineteenth and early twentieth centuries. The current form of the

'neurodevelopmental hypothesis' for the causation of schizophrenia was formulated in the 1980s (Lewis and Murray 1987). In brief, the neurodevelopmental hypothesis of schizophrenia postulates that an early (and fixed) lesion to the brain causes neural networks to be abnormally constituted. Psychotic symptoms are generated subsequently in early adulthood when these compromised neural networks fail to mature effectively or fail to cope with increased cognitive and social demands. The neurodevelopmental hypothesis has been criticised for its lack of specificity and its lack of a mechanism to explain progression from early neurodevelopmental abnormality to later onset of symptoms. Nevertheless, accumulating epidemiological evidence is compatible with a neurodevelopmental aetiology, as reviewed in this chapter.

Premorbid abnormalities in schizophrenia

NEUROLOGICAL DYSFUNCTION

Neurological abnormalities are consistently found in people with schizophrenia (Griffiths et al. 1998) and are associated with functional consequences, such as reduced academic achievement. Neurological abnormalities are an inherent part of the schizophrenia phenotype and are not accounted for by medication with neuroleptics (Malla et al. 1995). There is much evidence that they are present before the illness presents (Karp et al. 2001). For example, children who later develop schizophrenia have an increased incidence of so-called soft neurological abnormalities, along with deficits in social functioning and cognitive performance (Cannon et al. 1997). A systematic review reported that abnormalities in motor coordination and sequencing, sensory integration and developmental reflexes were already present in first-episode psychosis (Dazzan and Murray 2002). These neurological abnormalities are interpreted as evidence for early brain lesions with delayed motor development. Midline facial and dermatoglyphic anomalies are also evidence of early disrupted neurological development in fetal life.

BEHAVIOUR AND COGNITION

Neuropsychological and behavioural impairment in multiple domains have also been associated with schizophrenia and evidence suggests they are present prior to onset of the illness (e.g. Keshavan et al. 2005), although the onset and course of these deficits remains unclear. Cognitive deficits, language delay, social maladjustment, suspiciousness and relationship difficulties in childhood have also been associated with later development of schizophrenia (Cannon et al. 2001, 2004). Cognitive and behavioural deficits may thus be manifest 10–15 years before the first symptoms of psychosis develop.

BRAIN STRUCTURE

Structural imaging in schizophrenia, using computed tomography and magnetic resonance imaging, has demonstrated brain abnormalities, the earliest and most replicated finding being enlargement of the lateral ventricles (Johnstone et al. 1976). There are also more subtle volumetric irregularities of various regions, including the hippocampus, frontal cortex and subcortical structures (Wright et al. 2000, Boos et al. 2007), along with abnormalities in gyrification (Vogeley et al. 2001) and corresponding changes in microcirculation

(Lewis and Sweet 2009). These anomalies have been shown at first onset of illness and also in individuals at 'high risk' of schizophrenia (i.e. those with a family history in a first-degree relative) (Sowell et al. 2000). Functional neuroimaging studies, using positron emission tomography and single-photon emission computed tomography, have further highlighted disruptions in neural connectivity, particularly those associated with dopamine dysregulation (Urban and Abi-Dargham 2010). Future studies are set to assess dysregulation in non-dopaminergic networks such as glutamatergic and GABA-ergic pathways.

DEVELOPMENTAL ECTODERMAL ABNORMALITIES

Other replicated findings in schizophrenia are minor physical anomalies (MPAs) and alterations of dermatoglyphic patterns (Ekerot 1990, Fananas et al. 1996, Bramon et al. 2005), typically total finger ridge and total a–b ridge counts. These are minor aberrations of ectodermal development, probably arising in the first or second trimesters of pregnancy. They have been interpreted as an indication of subtly altered development, which may also be represented in other organs of ectodermal origin—principally the central nervous system. Griffiths et al. (1998) found that MPAs were increased in non-familial (sporadic) patients with schizophrenia, rather than in patients with a strong family history (i.e. a strong genetic loading). This raises the possibility that MPAs may be associated with environmental factors acting to perturb development, rather than inherent genetic factors. Associations between a–b dermatoglyphic abnormalities in schizophrenia, obstetric complications and cerebral structural measures are reported (Van Os et al. 2000, Bramon et al. 2005).

Epidemiology of schizophrenia

BIRTH COMPLICATIONS

Many studies have suggested that people who develop schizophrenia experienced a higher rate of 'obstetric complications' at or before birth (Rosso et al. 2000, Abel and Morgan 2011). Hypoxia-related complications include acute hypoxic events, such as prolapse of the umbilical cord, or other causes of intra-natal hypoxia or chronic hypoxia associated with placental abnormalities, i.e. pre-eclampsia. Some propose a linear relationship between the number of hypoxic incidents and subsequent risk of illness (Cannon et al. 2004). However, many use stratifications which fail to distinguish or inaccurately categorise these obstetric complications' into events with disparate mechanisms.

With a focus on perinatal events, Geddes et al. (1999) reported significant associations between schizophrenia and preterm birth (<37 weeks), premature rupture of membranes and resuscitation of the fetus. Traditionally, in the psychiatric literature, little consideration has been given to disentangling effects of early versus late preterm birth (which may have very different causes and consequences), or poor fetal growth and preterm birth, which can be confounders and co-occur. Allin et al. (2004) assessed very preterm (<34 weeks) and very low birthweight (<2kg) high-risk infants. They suggested that very immature and sick neonates are at risk of brain lesions that compromise their neurological development. In the Helsinki High-Risk (HR) Study, pregnant women and their offspring (Suvisaari et al. 2012) were studied alongside matched pregnancies born in the same hospital. Women admitted with a psychotic disorder before birth showed no increase in incidence of obstetric complications as previously described. However, from this large Finnish registry, three obstetric complications were associated with future schizophrenia risk: pregnancy-related in utero maternal infection, gestational hypertension and, most commonly, placental abnormalities. This is consistent with our own, more recent study in a Scandinavian population cohort (Gunn Eide et al. 2013) discussed later in this chapter.

Studies which implicate placental function in the aetio-pathogenesis of neurodevelopmental disorder (Abel 2004) are increasingly finding favour. Bonnin et al. (2011) described disruptions to the placental serotonin synthetic pathway, considered as crucial for forebrain development in the first and early second trimester of pregnancy.

MATERNAL VIRAL INFECTION

Maternal influenza during the first trimester has been associated with an increased risk of schizophrenia in offspring as adult. Methodological problems with the older literature make conclusions less reliable: thus, original studies used ecological, population level exposure to infections during periods of influenza epidemic. Women were considered as 'exposed' if they were pregnant during the epidemic period rather than by serological diagnosis. Furthermore, estimation of trimester of exposure was notoriously inaccurate in earlier cohorts before ultrasound was routinely used to date pregnancies. Thus, using Finnish birth records, Mednick et al. (1988) famously reported that individuals in utero from the second trimester during the 1957 influenza epidemic were at increased risk of developing schizophrenia later in life. Wright et al. (1995) proposed that influenza in the second trimester may act to increase the likelihood of obstetric complications, thus raising the risk of schizophrenia through perinatal hypoxic brain damage. Many studies attempted to replicate the results of Mednick et al. (1988) and both positive and negative findings have been reported. Brown et al. (2000) studied a large prospective birth cohort in which data concerning infections during pregnancy were available from medical records. They reported that second trimester exposure to respiratory infections was associated with an increased risk of schizophrenia spectrum disorder. Subsequently, the same group (Brown et al. 2004) examined serological evidence of maternal influenza infection in relation to psychotic disorders in the offspring in a small birth cohort. They reported that exposure to influenza in the first trimester and the first half of the second trimester, was associated with a sevenfold increase in schizophrenia risk.

As well as influenza, other viral infections, for example, cytomegalovirus, herpes and rubella, as well as bacterial upper urinary tract and respiratory infections, also confer some risk (Sørensen et al. 2009). In a cohort of offspring of mothers with serologically confirmed clinical rubella, 20% were subsequently diagnosed with schizophrenia, corresponding to a 10- to 20-fold increase (Brown et al. 2001). Maternal cytokine levels in mid-gestation, particularly IL-8 and TNF-a (but not IL-6 and Il-1b), are also associated with increased risk of psychosis among offspring, coupling infection with inflammation (Buka et al. 2001, Brown et al. 2004). Although intrauterine infection is one of the most common causes of abnormal fetal growth, no study has yet addressed the possibility that the infection–schizophrenia association is confounded by adverse effects upon feto-placental function.

URBANICITY

Many studies have shown an association between schizophrenia and being born/raised in an urban environment. Mortensen et al. (1999) estimated that people born in Copenhagen had 2.4 times the risk of developing schizophrenia in adulthood than those born in rural Denmark. Urban dwelling may also influence risk: Pedersen and Mortensen (2001) used the Danish Register population database to assess the relationship between 'degree' of urbanicity and diagnoses of schizophrenia. They found that living for 5 years in a large city increased risk of schizophrenia 1.4-fold. They suggested that there were linear relationships between the size of the city, the length of time lived in it and the risk of developing schizophrenia. The aetiological factor(s) responsible for these findings remains to be elucidated, but it may interact with socio-economic status and exposure to respiratory viruses, both independently associated with preterm birth and schizophrenia. Eaton et al. (2000), from the same group, suggested that the urbanicity effect in schizophrenia is not mediated through obstetric complications, although their sample was too small to confirm a lack of interaction.

FAMINE IN PREGNANCY

At the end of the Second World War, in German-occupied areas of the Netherlands, a German blockade cut off food and fuel shipments from farm areas, causing a famine during the winter of 1944–1945, exacerbated by the unusually cold weather that year (Hunger Winter). Susser and Lin (1992) reported that the offspring of mothers exposed to this famine during the first trimester of pregnancy had an elevated risk of developing schizophrenia in adulthood. This effect was found in female rather than male offspring. The Chinese famine of 1959–1961 was similarly studied by St Clair et al. (2005), who reported rates of schizophrenia compared among those born before, during and after the famine years. They reported a –one- to twofold excess risk of schizophrenia in those exposed to famine in utero. St Clair et al. were also able to show that birth rates decreased during the famine by 80% and that this nadir coincided with increased schizophrenia risk. This suggests that women conceiving may have been in better maternal condition than most or that they were not as nutritionally compromised (again records of individual nutritional intake were sparse). We still cannot distinguish whether famine influences outcomes through micronutrient lack, caloric deficit or most likely a combination of both.

Perhaps one of the most interesting more recent findings, relating to these famine studies, is the epigenetic effects reported by Heijmans et al. (2008) who found less DNA methylation in the IGF2 genes of exposed compared with unexposed same-sex siblings, six decades later. This was confined to those exposed in peri-conceptional periods rather than late pregnancy. Individuals with schizophrenia, who were in utero during the Hunger Winter, showed reduced brain volumes (Hulshoff-Pol et al. 2000). Brain structural abnormalities, particularly white matter hyper intensities, were also found in otherwise undiagnosed individuals, equally exposed to the famine in the first trimester. Such individuals have an increased risk of developing abnormalities of glucose tolerance in adulthood, unlike their peers born in the preceding year (Ravelli et al. 1998).

MATERNAL STRESS

Evidence for an association between antenatal maternal stress and perinatal outcomes such as preterm labour and fetal growth restriction is relatively robust (Mulder et al. 2002, Dole et al. 2003). Accumulating evidence from animal studies suggests that prenatal maternal stress may lead to reprogramming of neuroendocrine systems in the offspring, with subsequent effects on behaviour (Suomi 1997). In humans, Erickson et al. (2001) prospectively examined maternal hypothalamic–pituitary–adrenal (HPA) axis hormones, demographic factors and perception of stress in a small cohort of women at 7–23 weeks and 27–37 weeks of pregnancy. Early pregnancy maternal HPA axis parameters were not a good predictor of preterm birth, although maternal free corticotrophin levels in late pregnancy were significantly higher in women delivering preterm. The best predictors of preterm birth were previous preterm delivery, low socio-economic status and low level of education.

Some cognitive and brain developmental outcomes are also described following ante-natal maternal stress (Buss et al. 2010, 2012). However, its association with more severe mental illness risk in offspring is less consistent. The methodologically strongest studies to date report that offspring of mothers exposed to severe psychological stress antenatally or during the first 2 years of childhood have no increased risk of schizophrenia, non-affective psychosis or bipolar disorder (Abel et al. 2014, Class et al. 2014).

BIRTHWEIGHT

Lower birthweight (LBW: defined by the World Health Organization as <2500g) among individuals who later develop schizophrenia has been one of the most consistent findings (Abel et al. 2010). Moreover, smaller head circumference and being small for gestational age have also been associated with schizophrenia, pointing to an underlying mechanism of fetal growth restriction (Sacker et al. 1996, McNeil et al. 2000, Gunn Eide et al. 2013). It has been suggested that intrauterine growth restriction may be particularly related to early-onset schizophrenia in males (Gunnell et al. 2003). Wahlbeck et al. (2001) proposed that LBW, small size and reduced volume of the placenta at birth have a linear association with schizophrenia risk. However, using absolute birthweight as the predictor variable for schizophrenia risk is likely to be an inaccurate estimate of the effect of abnormal fetal growth (Wilcox 2001). Although earlier smaller studies, such as Gunnell et al. (2003), examined the association between birthweight, adult height and schizophrenia, with a reported association between heavier birthweight (>4kg) and increased risk, the largest definitive study of this association found no effect of high birthweight per se (Abel et al. 2010). In this study, we identified a general association between birthweight and risk of schizophrenia across the whole birthweight range, not just that less than 2500g. We went on to assess the effects of deviance from normal fetal growth (Gunn Eide et al. 2013) and suggest that, indeed, deviance from growth potential in utero may be more important than absolute size or birthweight as a predictor of schizophrenia in adulthood. In addition, we found the same relationship existed for other mental disorders such as bipolar disorder and non-psychotic disorders, although the effects were smaller. We therefore proposed a common mechanism leading to these different disorders, depending on genetic or environmental effects. In establishing a link between birthweight and development of psychiatric disorders in adulthood, we now discuss its possible aetiology.

Birthweight and health associations

BIRTHWEIGHT, GESTATIONAL AGE, SEX AND NEURODEVELOPMENTAL OUTCOMES

Abnormal fetal growth is well established as a significant cause of morbidity and mortality among newborn infants. Birthweight is significantly associated with global cognitive ability at age 8 years, through adolescence and into early adulthood, independent of social background (Gorman and Pollitt 1992). As proposed, these associations are evident across the normal birthweight range (>2.5–4kg) and so not accounted exclusively by LBW (Richards et al. 2001). Adjustment for gestational age, parity and socio-economic status, also fail to remove this effect.

This has also been examined in twin studies where difference in IQ within same sex pairs is accounted for by differences in birthweight. This effect is seen only in males (Shenkin et al. 2001). Johnson and Breslau (2000) reported that specific maths and reading disability occurred in girls and boys aged 11 years in both the LBW and normal birthweight ranges, although the significance was confined to LBW boys. The Surveillance of Cerebral Palsy in Europe collaboration of European Cerebral Palsy Registers assessed birthweight and gestation of a large cohort of children compared with reference standards for the normal spread of gestation and weight-for-gestational-age at birth. They reported an excess of cerebral palsy in both light- and heavy-for-gestation infants, in a reversed J-shaped pattern around an apparent optimal gestational weight (Jarvis et al. 2003).

Although family characteristics which cannot be measured may confound results somewhat, cognitive ability, as measured by IQ, is consistently found to relate directly to fetal growth across the normal birthweight range (Richards et al. 2001). At the higher and lower ends of the birthweight spectrum, the relationship is more complex particularly because of variation in gestational age. Few studies examine changes in cognitive ability by gestational age and it is often assumed that children born at term are homogeneous with respect to long-term cognitive and neurodevelopmental outcomes. Generally studies have been too small to examine variation in cognitive ability by each week of gestation among children born at or beyond 37 completed weeks. Amongst preterm infants, there is no evidence of a threshold effect: risk of a reduction in IQ declines steadily with advancing gestational age up to 37 weeks. However, there is a lack of information on whether beyond this and across early post-term periods (41–43 weeks of gestation), IQ tends to improve or to decline. There is even less information about risks of intellectual disability associated with later post-term (44–45 weeks). Because gestational age after term can be manipulated clinically by induction of labour, a simple clinical intervention could lead to prevention of disability. In male Norwegian conscripts, intelligence scores fell in those born from 41 to 44 weeks of gestation (Eide et al. 2007). More recently, using data from a 2005 school census in Scotland, Mackay et al. (2010) assessed risk of special educational need across a broader spectrum of gestational age where special educational need included intellectual disabilities, incorporating dyslexia, dyspraxia, autism, Asperger syndrome and attention-deficit–hyperactivity disorder, as well as children with physical disabilities that may affect learning. They reported a very strong association with extreme preterm delivery and, although the risk steadily declined with increasing gestational age up to 40–41 weeks, it began to increase in post-term deliveries. However, even in this relatively large sample ($n = 407,503$), they did not have enough power to assess risks specifically for post-term infants for individual weeks of gestational age or to examine specific educational need individually.

In a far smaller cohort, Yang et al. (2010) examined children at age 6.5 years born at term with normal weight. Compared with the score for those born at 39–41 weeks, the full-scale IQ score was 1.7 points lower (95% confidence interval (CI): –2.7, –0.7) in children born at 37 weeks and 0.4 points lower (95% CI: –1.1, 0.02) at 38 weeks. In post-term children, there was 0.5-points lower (95% CI: –2.6, 1.6) score at 42 weeks and 0.6 points lower (95% CI: –15.1, 3.1) at 43 weeks; they did not look at gestational age beyond 43 weeks.

Our recent findings suggest increased risk of intellectual disability with autism in post-term infants who were growth restricted (OR 2.72 95% CI: 1.76–4.18) (Abel et al. 2013).

The well-described link between fetal growth and variations in cognitive ability have not been replicated in sibling analyses (Losh et al. 2011) which gives some weight to the idea that effects might be because of unmeasured family characteristics. Relationships between gestational age, fetal growth and cognitive ability are undoubtedly complex. Cognitive ability is such an important predictor of many life outcomes that more detailed understanding is needed to inform better obstetric care and child outcomes.

Male vulnerability

In most abnormal neurodevelopmental outcomes, males are consistently shown to be the 'weaker' sex. Newborn males have higher mortality rates than females at all gestational ages and are at greater risk of complications such as cerebral palsy (Sizun et al. 1998). Males have a higher prevalence of developmental and learning difficulties (Johnson and Breslau 2000) and schizophrenia (Aleman et al. 2003). They are also more prone to the perinatal brain injury associated with LBW and pre- and postterm birth (Shankaran et al. 1996) and are more likely than girls to show later neurological and cognitive impairment and learning difficulties (Hindmarsh et al. 2000). This idea, that the early post/perinatal origins of schizophrenia are more prevalent in males than females, is firmly supported by animal studies. Given the general significance of birthweight and gestational age to neurodevelopmental outcomes, including schizophrenia risk, the notion of hypoxic-ischaemic damage, in utero or postnatally, may be less important than previously thought (van Erp et al. 2002). The following section therefore explores alternative aetiological mechanisms, attempting to account for this excess male incidence.

Abnormal fetal growth, cardiovascular disease and insulin resistance

Apart from abnormal neurodevelopmental outcomes, abnormal fetal growth is also associated with poor health in adulthood due to a constellation of disorders referred to as 'Syndrome X'. This includes hypertension, coronary artery disease and type 2 diabetes (Gluckman and Harding 1997). Reduced insulin sensitivity or insulin resistance is a common feature of these diseases and is overt, before the diseases manifest. Fetal adaptation to an adverse intrauterine environment may involve altered programming of growth and endocrine pathways, leading to permanent metabolic changes, including reduced insulin sensitivity (Barker 1995). It is suggested that many of the later adult sequelae could be explained as a consequence of this change (Hofman et al. 1997).

The parents of LBW offspring, especially the fathers, show an increased risk of type 2 diabetes. Moreover, people with sporadic schizophrenia (with no family history) are not only more likely to have been LBW themselves, as previously discussed, but are also more prone to develop insulin resistance and type 2 diabetes, as are their unaffected relatives (Ryan et al. 2003). This points to a mechanistic overlap between the control of fetal growth and insulin sensitivity and cause of schizophrenia (Abel 2004). Hattersley and Tooke (1999) proposed the common mechanism to be genetic, suggesting that a large component of variation in fetal weight may be explained by genetic control in the fetus of glucose sensing, insulin secretion and particularly insulin resistance.

GENOMIC IMPRINTING AND THE CONFLICT HYPOTHESIS

Genomic imprinting is a mammalian parent-of-origin-dependent form of gene regulation and a notable exception to Mendelian laws of inheritance. The most frequently studied form of such gene regulation is DNA methylation and is typically associated with chromatin condensation through the binding of methyl-CpG binding proteins and recruitment of proteins involved in chromatin modification. These ultimately lead to transcriptional silencing or genomic imprinting. DNA methylation regulates genomically imprinted genes through differential marking of the parental alleles during two epigenetic reprogramming events in early pregnancy; in gametogenesis, when methylation is erased and re-established to reflect the sex of the individual in which the developing gametes reside and after fertilisation, when the maternal and paternal pronuclei undergo demethylation and subsequent remethylation that will help guide germ layer specification and tissue differentiation. Imprinting, therefore, marks a subset of mammalian genes for allelic preference or, less commonly in humans, for mono-allelic expression and is responsible for the differential contributions of maternal and paternal genomes in mammals.

Most imprinted genes occur in clusters on the genome (e.g. chromosomes 7, 11, 15) and play a critical role in embryonic growth, CNS growth, social cognition and behavioural development, as well as cancer susceptibility. Imprinting evolved with the advent of mammalian (placentally dependent) live birth and divergence in imprinting may have coincided with increasing brain size (Killian et al. 2001). Insulin growth factors (IGFs) were the first imprinted genes to be identified and they are now known to be crucial for placental development (see Chapter 3) along with other imprinted genes (Constancia et al. 2002). Placental-specific IGF-II is a major modulator of placental growth. The IGF-II gene is paternally expressed in the fetus and the placenta (Constancia et al. 2002). Deletion of the paternally expressed IGF-II, Peg1/Mest, Peg3 or Ins1/ins2 genes results in intrauterine growth restriction, whereas deletion of the maternally expressed IGF-II or H19 genes, or overexpression of paternal IGF-II gene results in fetal overgrowth. Other imprinted genes are involved in the organisation and behaviour of placental cell types. Because of their effects on placental structure and physiology, imprinted genes could also control fetal growth by acting in the placenta to influence the supply of nutrients to the fetus (Reik et al. 2003).

The genetic conflict hypothesis predicts that paternally expressed genes acting in the placenta will aim to extract more resources from the mother to enhance fetal growth, whereas maternally expressed genes will aim to restrain fetal growth to conserve resources for future offspring. Constancia et al. (2002) described evidence in support of this theory: IGF-II and other imprinted genes, such as Peg 1, appear to control both the placental supply of and the fetal demand for, maternal nutrients. Studies have examined whether variation in these parental alleles might explain some of the variability in fetal weight in humans. One such gene polymorphism is the insulin gene variable number of tandem repeat polymorphism (INS-VNTR). The INS-VNTR lies upstream of the insulin (INS) and IGF-II genes and is associated with variations in the transcription of IGFs. Dunger et al. (1998) reported that variation in these allele polymorphisms is associated with variation in birthweight, but Mitchell et al. (2004) failed to replicate these findings or to support a parent-of-origin effect. Other groups have examined promoter polymorphisms in the IGF-I gene and reported that these are associated with reductions in head circumference and persisting short stature in children born LBW or small for gestational age (Vaessen et al. 2002). Fetal genes controlling glucose sensing also appear relevant, as Hattersley et al. (1998) found that mutations in the glucokinase gene result in a reduction in birthweight.

Genomic imprinting and schizophrenia

Accumulating evidence suggests that an organism's ability to adapt to early environmental cues, such as in utero exposure to maternal stressors or cigarette smoking, are realised through changes in the methylation patterns perhaps particularly in differentially methylated regions (DMRs) of imprinted genes (Feng et al. 2010, Kota and Feil 2010). This mechanism provides the organism with early epigenetic plasticity. Some maternal exposures, which have been related epidemiologically to risk of neurodevelopmental disorder, including schizophrenia in later life, have been shown, by some (Heijmans et al. 2008 pregnancy-related famine) but not all (Waterland et al. 2010), to be associated in adults with methylation differences at the IGF2 DMR, between individuals exposed to environmental stimuli such as nutrient challenges. This suggests that this DMR is a reasonable epigenetic 'biosensor' for evaluating early environmental exposures (Hoyo et al. 2009). Indeed, it has been suggested that methylation shifts at sequences regulating genomic imprinting can serve as archives of the periconceptional and prenatal environment (Mathers, 2007, Heijmans et al. 2008, Hoyo et al. 2009). However, to date, studies show inconsistency in the patterns of mehylation associated with environmental exposures. Thus, Murphy et al. (2012) found that maternal cigarette smoking increased methylation at the IGF2DMR, whereas the Dutch famine studies found hypomethylation at the IGF2 DMR following maternal caloric restriction in utero (Heijmans et al. 2008). In a study of 17-month-old children, folic acid improved a hypomethylated IGF2 DMR, presumably restoring genomic imprinting (Steegers-Theunissen et al. 2009). These findings were not confirmed in a Gambian rural community conceived during the nutritionally challenging rainy season (Waterland et al. 2010).

Imprinting may be a polymorphic trait in humans. This is of particular interest as the neuropathological abnormalities, 'characteristic' of schizophrenia, show marked overlap with normal brain structural heterogeneity in the population and ventricle–brain ratio is normally distributed within schizophrenia (Harrison 1999). These features are compatible with the involvement of a process whose role is to regulate normal fetal growth and which is polymorphically expressed, such as imprinting.

Some studies have also shown that methylation changes at DMR genes are sex-dependent. Thus, Murphy et al. (2012) report maternal cigarette smoking differentially alters IGF2-regulating methylation in male children only. Interestingly, the birth-to-placental weight ratio is greater in male than in female infants and greatest in growth-restricted males (Edwards et al. 2000). Since males have relatively smaller placentae, factors that compromise placental function (including cigarette smoking) are likely to have greater impact on male brain growth. Sex-differentiated mechanisms may in part explain the greater prevalence of developmental disorders and neurodevelopmental schizophrenia in males. Reduction in neuronal size is regionally specific in schizophrenic brains, suggesting that whatever is responsible for the neurodevelopmental abnormality has some specificity. Neocortical areas, such as the prefrontal cortex, are last to mature and therefore may be more vulnerable to growth abnormalities. Of note, in the neurogenetic disorder Angelman syndrome, which is thought to be associated with inappropriate imprinting of chromosome 15q11-13, anomalies of cortical growth occur, including cortical atrophy, microencephaly and ventricular dilatation (for a review, see Davies et al. 2001).

Abnormalities of imprinting have also been described in disorders of abnormal growth control such as tumours. For example, a lack of imprinting, or overexpression of paternal IGF2, has been described in gigantism associated with Wilm's tumours (Vu et al. 2003). If schizophrenia were associated with excessive imprinting, or an under-expression of imprinted genes (effective deletion of an imprinted gene), one might expect opposite effects, i.e. less tumorigenesis and reduced growth. There is some evidence that this is the case. Relatives of people with schizophrenia are less likely than the general population to develop cancer; people with schizophrenia have been reported to suffer both more and less cancer, although a population of patients with schizophrenia controlled for smoking and socioeconomic factors has yet to be studied (Jablensky and Lawrence 2001). Deletion of paternally expressed IGF-II results in reduced fetal growth and insulin resistance in later life (Ozanne and Hales 1999), both of which are characteristics of schizophrenic phenotypes (Ryan et al. 2003).

Abnormal imprinting is consistent with the parent-of-origin and paternal age effects observed in schizophrenia. Maternal schizophrenia may be associated with inherited abnormalities of imprinting (e.g. loci of imprinted genes may be adjacent to loci relevant to schizophrenia) or with environmental factors (reduced maternal resources or increased maternal environmental stressors) that promote changes in imprinting such as reduction of paternally expressed IGF-II. Abnormalities of paternally expressed IGF-II may also be more likely to occur in older parents. Season-of-birth effects in schizophrenia might also be explained by seasonal alterations in IGF expression or regulation and placental development as reported in sheep. However, if the developmental disruption associated with schizophrenia is linked to methylation changes in IGF2, the direction of altered imprinting is unclear. As adults, Dutch famine survivors (who show excess risk for schizophrenia at least in males) are also at significantly higher risk of neurological disorders, obesity in early and late adulthood, breast cancer, infertility and metabolic disorders that include type 2 diabetes and dyslipidemia and many of these outcomes are also more common in schizophrenia sufferers and their relatives (see Abel 2004, Murphy et al. 2012). Nevertheless, studies have shown both increased and decreased methylation at IGF2 within affected individuals.

Placenta and autism spectrum disorders

Autism spectrum disorders (ASDs) are genetically and phenomenologically linked to schizophrenia. In particular, individuals with ASD and schizophrenia show abnormalities of social cognition and are more likely than healthy individuals to have intellectual disability. ASDs have recently been linked to placental aberrations (Walker et al. 2013). In this case, placental differences manifest histologically through an increase in placental trophoblast inclusions (Walker et al. 2013). The proposed commonality is one of increased cellular growth and tissue folding in both affected placentae and adolescent brain. Some evidence suggests that ASD may be associated with preterm brain growth in the first year of life (Chawarska et al. 2011). Microscopic and macroscopic evidence of abnormal brain folding has also been reported (Nordahl et al. 2007). However, further confirmation is required. Our own recent population study found evidence that deviance in fetal growth at both extremes (high and low fetal growth) was associated with increased risk of ASD. We also reported an independent effect of preterm birth. Overall, risks were highest for ASD and intellectual disability in growth-restricted infants, who were also postmature (Abel et al. 2013).

Future directions

Abnormal placental function and dysregulation of fetal growth are increasingly considered in the aetiology of rare neurodevelopmental disorders like schizophrenia and autism with implications for our understanding of the origins of cognitive ability. This generates a wealth of new research avenues. One of the more exciting considers the role of aberrant imprinting in genes common to fetal growth and brain growth. Animal knockouts and knock-ins are improving our understanding of the links between imprinting, placental function and neurodevelopment. Future large database epidemiology may allow further exploration of how the effects of epigenetic disruption are influenced by maternal versus paternal genes, in female versus male offspring and by environmental factors. As markers of placental function become available, population-based cord blood samples may allow study of such effects in large cohorts of women at risk.

REFERENCES

Abel KM (2004) Fetal origins of schizophrenia: Testable hypotheses of genetic and environmental influences. *Br J Psychiatry* 184: 383–385. doi: http://dx.doi.org/10.1192/bjp.184.5.383.

Abel KM, Heuvelman H, Jorgensen L et al. (2014) Does prenatal or childhood severe psychological stress increase the risk of subsequent psychosis? A Swedish national population cohort. *BMJ* 348: f7679.

Abel KM, Morgan VA (2011) Women and mothers with mental illness, and their children (Chapter 19). In: Tsuang MT, Tohen M, Jones PJ, editors. *Psychiatric Epidemiology*, 3rd ed. John Wiley & Sons, New York.

Abel KM, Svensson A, Dal H et al. (2013) Deviance fetal growth and autism spectrum disorder. *Am J Psychiatry* 170: 391–398.

Abel KM, Wicks S, Susser E et al. (2010) Birth weight, schizophrenia and adult mental disorder: Is risk confined to the smallest babies? *Arch Gen Psychiatry* 67: 923–930. doi: http://dx.doi.org/10.1001/archgenpsychiatry.2010.100.

Aleman A, Kahn R, Selten JP (2003) Sex differences in risk of schizophrenia: Evidence from meta-analysis. *Arch Gen Psychiatry* 60: 565–571. doi: http://dx.doi.org/10.1001/archpsyc.60.6.565.

Allin M, Nosarti C, Rifkin L, Murray RM (2004) Brain plasticity and long term function after early cerebral insult: The example of very preterm birth. In: Keshavan M, Kennedy J, Murray RM, editors. *Neurodevelopment and Schizophrenia*, 89–107. Cambridge: Cambridge University Press.

Barker DJ (1995) Intrauterine programming of adult disease. *Mol Med Today* 1(9): 418–423. doi: http://dx.doi.org/10.1016/s1357-4310(95)90793-9.

Bonnin A, Goeden N, Chen K et al. (2011) A transient placental source of serotonin for the fetal forebrain. *Nature* 472(7343): 347–350. doi: http://dx.doi.org/10.1038/nature09972.

Boos HB, Aleman A, Cahn W, Hulshoff Pol H, Kahn RS (2007) Brain volumes in relatives of patients with schizophrenia: A meta-analysis. *Arch Gen Psychiatry* 64(3): 297–304. doi: http://dx.doi.org/10.1001/archpsyc.64.3.297.

Bramon E, Walshe M, McDonald C et al. (2005) Dermatoglyphics and schizophrenia: A meta-analysis and investigation of the impact of obstetric complications upon a–b ridge count. *Schizophr Res* 75: 399–404. doi: http://dx.doi.org/10.1016/j.schres.2004.08.022.

Brown, AS, Begg, MD, Gravenstein S et al. (2004) Serologic evidence of prenatal influenza in the etiology of schizophrenia. *Arch Gen Psychiatry* 61: 774–780.

Brown AS, Cohen P, Harkavy-Friedman J et al. (2001) A.E. Bennett Research Award. Prenatal rubella, premorbid abnormalities, and adult schizophrenia. *Biol Psychiatry* 49(6): 473–486. doi: http://dx.doi.org/10.1016/s0006-3223(01)01068-x.

Brown AS, Schaefer CA, Wyatt RJ et al. (2000) Maternal exposure to respiratory infections and adult schizophrenia spectrum disorders: A prospective birth cohort study. *Schizophr Bull* 26: 287–295. doi: http://dx.doi.org/10.1093/oxfordjournals.schbul.a033453.

Buka SL, Tsuang MT, Torrey EF, Klebanoff MA, Wagner RL, Yolken RH (2001) Maternal cytokine levels during pregnancy and adult psychosis. *Brain Behav Immun* 15(4): 411–420. doi: http://dx.doi.org/10.1006/brbi.2001.0644.

Buss C, Davis EP, Muftuler LT, Head K, Sandman CA (2010) High pregnancy anxiety during mid-gestation is associated with decreased gray matter density in 6–9-year-old children. *Psychoneuroendocrinology* 35: 141–153. doi: http://dx.doi.org/10.1016/j.psyneuen.2009.07.010.

Buss C, Davis EP, Shahbaba B, Pruessner JC, Head K, Sandman CA (2012) Maternal cortisol over the course of pregnancy and subsequent child amygdala and hippocampus volumes and affective problems. *Proc Natl Acad Sci* 109: E1312–E1319. doi: http://dx.doi.org/10.1073/pnas.1201295109.

Cannon M, Dean K, Jones PB (2004) Early environmental risk factors for schizophrenia. In: Keshavan M, Kennedy J, Murray RM, editors. *Neurodevelopment and Schizophrenia*, 191–209. Cambridge: Cambridge University Press.

Cannon M, Jones P, Gilvarry C et al. (1997) Premorbid social functioning in schizophrenia and bipolar disorder: Similarities and differences. *Am J Psychiatry* 154: 1544–1550.

Cannon M, Walsh E, Hollis C et al. (2001) Predictors of later schizophrenia and affective psychosis among attendees at a child psychiatry department. *Br J Psychiatry* 178: 420–426. doi: http://dx.doi.org/10.1192/bjp.178.5.420.

Cardno AG, Marshall EJ, Coid B et al. (1999) Heritability estimates for psychotic disorders: The Maudsley twin psychosis series. *Arch Gen Psychiatry* 56: 162–168. doi: http://dx.doi.org/10.1001/archpsyc.56.2.162.

Chawarska K, Campbell D, Chen L, Shic F, Klin A, Chang J (2011) Early generalized overgrowth in boys with autism. *Arch Gen Psychiatry* 68(10): 1021–1031. doi: http://dx.doi.org/10.1001/archgenpsychiatry.2011.106.

Class QA, Abel KM, Khashan AS et al (2014) Offspring psychopathology following preconception, prenatal, and postnatal maternal bereavement stress. *Psychol Med* 44(1): 71–84. doi: http://dx.doi.org/10.1017/s0033291713000780.

Constancia M, Hemberger M, Hughes J et al. (2002) Placental-specific IGF-II is a major modulator of placental and fetal growth. *Nature* 417: 945–948. doi: http://dx.doi.org/10.1038/nature00819.

Davies W, Isles AR, Wilkinson LS (2001) Imprinted genes and mental dysfunction. *Trends Mol Med* 33: 428–435. doi: http://dx.doi.org/10.3109/07853890108995956.

Dazzan P, Murray RM (2002) Neurological soft signs in first-episode psychosis: A systematic review. *Br J Psychiatry* 181(Suppl 43): s50–s57. doi: http://dx.doi.org/10.1192/bjp.181.43.s50.

Doherty JL, O'Donovan MC, Owen MJ (2012) Recent genomic advances in schizophrenia. *Clin Genet* 81(2): 103–109. doi: http://dx.doi.org/10.1111/j.1399-0004.2011.01773.x.

Dole N, Savitz DA, Hertz-Picciotto I, Siega-Riz AM, McMahon MJ, Buekens P (2003) Maternal stress and preterm birth. *Am J Epidemiol* 157: 14–24. doi: http://dx.doi.org/10.1093/aje/kwf176.

Dunger DB, Ong KK, Huxtable SJ et al. (1998) Association of the INS VNTR with size at birth. ALSPAC Study Team. Avon Longitudinal Study of Pregnancy and Childhood. *Nat Genet* 19: 98–100. doi: http://dx.doi.org/10.1038/ng0598-98.

Eaton WW, Mortensen PB, Frydenberg M (2000) Obstetric factors, urbanization and psychosis. *Schizophr Res* 43: 117–123. doi: http://dx.doi.org/10.1016/s0920-9964(99)00152-8.

Edwards A, Megens A, Peek M, Wallace EM (2000) Sexual origins of placental dysfunction. *Lancet* 355: 203–204. doi: http://dx.doi.org/10.1016/s0140-6736(99)05061-8.

Eide MG, Moster D, Irgens L et al. (2013) Degree of fetal growth restriction associated with schizophrenia risk in a national cohort. *Psychol Med* 43(10): 2057–2066. doi: http://dx.doi.org/10.1017/s003329171200267x.

Eide MG, Oyen N, Skjaerven R, Bjerkedal T (2007) Associations of birth size, gestational age, and adult size with intellectual performance: Evidence from a cohort of Norwegian men. *Pediatr Res* 62: 636–642. doi: http://dx.doi.org/10.1203/pdr.0b013e31815586e9.

Ekerot CF (1990) The lateral reticular nucleus in the cat. VII. Excitatory and inhibitory projection from the ipsilateral forelimb tract (iF tract). *Exp Brain Res* 79(1): 120–128. doi: http://dx.doi.org/10.1007/bf00228880.

Erickson K, Thorsen P, Chrousos G et al. (2001) Preterm birth: Associated neuroendocrine, medical, and behavioural risk factors. *J Clin Endocrinol Metab* 86: 2544–2552.

Fananas L, van Os J, Hoyos C, McGrath J, Mellor CS, Murray R (1996) Dermatoglyphic a–b ridge count as a possible marker for developmental disturbance in schizophrenia: Replication in two samples. *Schizophr Res* 20: 307–314. doi: http://dx.doi.org/10.1016/0920-9964(95)00013-5.

Feng S, Cokus SJ, Zhang X et al. (2010) Conservation and divergence of methylation patterning in plants and animals. *Proc Natl Acad Sci USA* 107: 8689–8694. doi: http://dx.doi.org/10.1073/pnas.1002720107.

Geddes JR, Verdoux H, Takei N et al. (1999) Schizophrenia and complications of pregnancy and labor: An individual patient data meta-analysis. *Schizophr Bull* 25(3): 413–423. doi: http://dx.doi.org/10.1093/oxfordjournals.schbul.a033389.

Gluckman PD, Harding JE (1997) The physiology and pathophysiology of intrauterine growth retardation. *Horm Res* 48: 11–16. doi: http://dx.doi.org/10.1159/000191257.

Gorman KS, Pollitt E (1992) Relationship between weight and body proportionality at birth, growth during the first year of life, and cognitive development at 36, 48, and 60 months. *Infant Behav Develop* 15: 279–296. doi: http://dx.doi.org/10.1016/0163-6383(92)80001-b.

Griffiths TD, Sigmundsson T, Takei N, Rowe D, Murray RM (1998) Neurological soft signs in familial and sporadic schizophrenia. *Brain* 121: 191–203.

Gunnell D, Rasmussen F, Fouskakis D, Tynelius P, Harrison G (2003) Patterns of fetal and childhood growth and the development of psychosis in young males: A cohort study. *Am J Epidemiol* 158: 291–300. doi: http://dx.doi.org/10.1093/aje/kwg118.

Harrison PJ (1999) The neuropathology of schizophrenia: A critical review of the data and their interpretation. *Brain* 122: 593–624. doi: http://dx.doi.org/10.1093/brain/122.4.593.

Hattersley AT, Beards F, Ballantyne E, Appleton M, Harvey R, Ellard S (1998) Mutations in the glucokinase gene of the fetus result in reduced birth weight. *Nat Genet* 19: 268–270. doi: http://dx.doi.org/10.1038/953.

Hattersley AT, Tooke JE (1999) The fetal insulin hypothesis: An alternative explanation of the association of low birth weight with diabetes and vascular disease. *Lancet* 353: 1789–1792. doi: http://dx.doi.org/10.1016/s0140-6736(98)07546-1.

Heijmans BT, Tobi EW, Stein AD et al. (2008) Persistent epigenetic differences associated with prenatal exposure to famine in humans. *Proc Natl Acad Sci USA* 105(44): 17046–17049. doi: http://dx.doi.org/10.1073/pnas.0806560105.

118

Hindmarsh GJ, O'Callaghan MJ, Mohay HA, Rogers YM (2000) Gender differences in cognitive abilities at 2 years in ELBW infants. Extremely low birth weight. *Early Hum Dev* 60: 115–122. doi: http://dx.doi.org/10.1016/s0378-3782(00)00105-5.

Hofman PL, Cutfield WS, Robinson EM et al. (1997) Insulin resistance in short children with intrauterine growth retardation. *J Clin Endocrinol Metab* 82: 402–406. doi: http://dx.doi.org/10.1210/jcem.82.2.3752.

Hoyo C, Murphy SK, Jirtle RL (2009) Imprint regulatory elements as epigenetic biosensors of exposure in epidemiological studies. *J Epidemiol Community Health* 63: 683–684. doi: http://dx.doi.org/10.1136/jech.2009.090803.

Hulshoff Pol HE, Hoek HE, Susser E et al. (2000) Prenatal exposure to famine and brain morphology in schizophrenia. *Am J Psychiatry* 157: 1170–1172. doi: http://dx.doi.org/10.1176/appi.ajp.157.7.1170.

Jablensky A, Lawrence D (2001) Schizophrenia and cancer: Is there a need to invoke a protective gene? *Arch Gen Psychiatry* 58: 579–580. doi: http://dx.doi.org/10.1001/archpsyc.58.6.579.

Jarvis S, Glinianaia SV, Torrioli MG et al.; Surveillance of Cerebral Palsy in Europe (SCPE) collaboration of European Cerebral Palsy Registers (2003) Cerebral palsy and intrauterine growth in single births: European collaborative study. *Lancet* 362: 1106–1011. doi: http://dx.doi.org/10.1016/s0140-6736(03)14466-2.

Johnson EO, Breslau N (2000) Increased risk of learning disabilities in low birth weight boys at age 11 years. *Biol Psychiatry* 47: 490–500. doi: http://dx.doi.org/10.1016/s0006-3223(99)00223-1.

Johnstone EC, Crow TJ, Frith CD, Husband J, Kreel L (1976) Cerebral ventricular size and cognitive impairment in chronic schizophrenia. *Lancet* 308: 924–926. doi: http://dx.doi.org/10.1016/s0140-6736(76)90890-4.

Karp BI, Garvey M, Jacobsen LK et al. (2001) Abnormal neurologic maturation in adolescents with early-onset schizophrenia. *Am J Psychiatry* 158: 118–122. doi: http://dx.doi.org/10.1176/appi.ajp.158.1.118.

Keshavan MS, Diwadkar VA, Montrose DM, Rajarethinam R, Sweeney JA (2005) Premorbid indicators and risk for schizophrenia: A selective review and update. *Schizophr Res* 79: 45–57. doi: http://dx.doi.org/10.1016/j.schres.2005.07.004.

Killian JK, Nolan CM, Wylie AA et al. (2001) Divergent evolution in M6P/IGF2R imprinting from the Jurassic to the Quaternary. *Hum Mol Genet* 10: 1721–1728. doi: http://dx.doi.org/10.1093/hmg/10.17.1721.

Kota SK, Feil R (2010) Epigenetic transitions in germ cell development and meiosis. *Dev Cell* 19: 675–686. doi: http://dx.doi.org/10.1016/j.devcel.2010.10.009.

Lewis DA, Sweet RA (2009) Schizophrenia from a neural circuitry perspective: Advancing toward rational pharmacological therapies. *J Clin Invest* 119(4): 706–716. doi: http://dx.doi.org/10.1172/jci37335.

Lewis SW, Murray RM (1987) Obstetric complications, neurodevelopmental deviance and risk of schizophrenia. *J Psychiatr Res* 21: 413–421. doi: http://dx.doi.org/10.1016/0022-3956(87)90088-4.

Losh M, Esserman D, Anckarsater H, Sullivan PF, Lichtenstein P (2011) A twin study of low birth weight as a risk factor for autism. *Psychol Med* FirstView Article:1-12.

MacKay DF, Smith GCS, Dobbie R, Pell JP (2010) Gestational age at delivery and special educational need: Retrospective cohort study of 407,503 school children. *PLoS Med* 7(6): e1000289. doi: http://dx.doi.org/10.1371/journal.pmed.1000289.

McNeil TF, Cantor-Graae E, Ismail B (2000) Obstetric complications and congenital malformation in schizophrenia. *Brain Res Rev* 31(2–3): 166–178. doi: http://dx.doi.org/10.1016/s0165-0173(99)00034-x.

Malla AK, Norman RMG, Aguilar O, Carnahan H, Cortese L (1995) Relationship between movement planning and psychopathology profiles in schizophrenia. *Br J Psychiatry* 167: 211–215. doi: http://dx.doi.org/10.1192/bjp.167.2.211.

Mathers JC (2007) Early nutrition: Impact on epigenetics. *Forum Nutr* 60: 42–48. doi: http://dx.doi.org/10.1159/000107066.

Mednick SA, Machon RA, Huttunen MO, Bonett D (1988) Adult schizophrenia following prenatal exposure to an influenza epidemic. *Arch Gen Psychiatry* 45: 189–192. doi: http://dx.doi.org/10.1001/archpsyc.1988.01800260109013.

Mitchell SMS, Hattersley AT, Knight B et al. (2004) Lack of support for a role of the insulin gene variable number of tandem repeats minisatellite (INS-VNTR) locus in fetal growth or type 2 diabetes-related intermediate traits in United Kingdom populations. *J Clin Endocrinol Metab* 89: 310–317. doi: http://dx.doi.org/10.1210/jc.2003-030605.

Mortensen PB, Pedersen CB, Westergaard T et al. (1999) Effects of family history and place and season of birth on the risk of schizophrenia. *N Engl J Med* 340: 603–608. doi: http://dx.doi.org/10.1056/nejm199902253400803.

Mulder EJH, Robles de Medina PG, Huizink AC, Van den Bergh BRH, Buitelaar JK, Visser GHA (2002) Prenatal maternal stress: Effect on pregnancy and the (unborn) child. *Early Hum Dev* 70: 3–14. doi: http://dx.doi.org/10.1016/s0378-3782(02)00075-0.

Murphy SK, Adigun A, Huang Z et al. (2012) Gender-specific methylation differences in relation to prenatal exposure to cigarette smoke. *Gene* 494(1): 36–43. doi: http://dx.doi.org/10.1016/j.gene.2011.11.062.

Nordahl CW, Dierker D, Mostafavi I et al. (2007) Cortical folding abnormalities in autism revealed by surface-based morphometry. *J Neurosci* 27(43): 11725–11735. doi: http://dx.doi.org/10.1523/jneurosci.0777-07.2007.

Ozanne SE, Hales CN (1999) The long-term consequences of intra-uterine protein malnutrition for glucose metabolism. *Proc Nutr Soc* 58: 615–619. doi: http://dx.doi.org/10.1017/s0029665199000804.

Pedersen CB, Mortensen PB (2001) Family history, place and season of birth as risk factors for schizophrenia in Denmark: A replication and reanalysis. *Br J Psychiatry* 179: 46–52. doi: http://dx.doi.org/10.1192/bjp.179.1.46.

Ravelli AC, van der Meulen JH, Michels RP et al. (1998) Glucose tolerance in adults after prenatal exposure to famine. *Lancet* 351: 173–177. doi: http://dx.doi.org/10.1016/s0140-6736(97)07244-9.

Reik W, Constancia M, Fowden A et al. (2003) Regulation of supply and demand for maternal nutrients in mammals by imprinted genes. *J Physiol* 547: 35–44.

Richards M, Hardy R, Kuh D, Wadsworth MEJ (2001) Birth weight and cognitive function in the British 1946 birth cohort: Longitudinal population based study. *BMJ* 322: 199–203. doi: http://dx.doi.org/10.1136/bmj.322.7280.199.

Rosso IM, Cannon TD, Huttunen T, Huttunen MO, Lonnqvist J, Gasperoni TL (2000) Obstetric risk factors for early-onset schizophrenia in a Finnish birth cohort. *Am J Psychiatry* 157: 801–807. doi: http://dx.doi.org/10.1176/appi.ajp.157.5.801.

Ryan MCM, Collins P, Thakore JH (2003) Impaired fasting glucose tolerance in first-episode, drug-naïve patients with schizophrenia. *Am J Psychiatry* 160: 284–289. doi: http://dx.doi.org/10.1176/appi.ajp.160.2.284.

Sacker A, Done DJ, Crow TJ (1996) Obstetric complications in children born to parents with schizophrenia: A meta-analysis of case-control studies. *Psychol Med* 26(2): 279–287. doi: http://dx.doi.org/10.1017/s003329170003467x.

Shankaran S, Bauer C, Bain R, Wright L, Zachary J (1996) Prenatal and perinatal risk and protective factors for neonatal intracranial hemorrhage. National Institute of Child Health and Human Development Neonatal Research Network. *Arch Pediatr Adolesc Med* 150: 491–497. doi: http://dx.doi.org/10.1001/archpedi.1996.02170300045009.

Shenkin SD, Starr JM, Pattie A, Rush MA, Whalley LJ, Deary IJ (2001) Birth weight and cognitive function at age 11 years: The Scottish Mental Survey 1932. *Arch Dis Child* 85: 189–196. doi: http://dx.doi.org/10.1136/adc.85.3.189.

Sizun J, Le Pommelet C, Lemoine M et al. (1998) Neuro-intellectual prognosis at school age for 62 children born with gestational age of under 32 weeks. *Arch Pediatr* 5: 139–144.

Sorensen HJ, Mortensen EL, Reinisch JM, Mednick SA (2009) Association between prenatal exposure to bacterial infection and risk of schizophrenia. *Schizophr Bull* 35(3): 631–637. doi: http://dx.doi.org/10.1093/schbul/sbn121.

Sowell ER, Levitt J, Thompson PM et al. (2000) Brain abnormalities in early-onset schizophrenia spectrum disorder observed with statistical parametric mapping of structural magnetic resonance images. *Am J Psychiatry* 157: 1475–1484. doi: http://dx.doi.org/10.1176/appi.ajp.157.9.1475.

St Clair D, Xu M, Wang P et al. (2005) Rates of adult schizophrenia following prenatal exposure to the Chinese famine of 1959–1961. *JAMA* 294: 557–562. doi: http://dx.doi.org/10.1001/jama.294.5.557.

Steegers-Theunissen RP, Obermann-Borst SA, Kremer D et al. (2009) Periconceptional maternal folic acid use of 400 μg per day is related to increased methylation of the *IGF2* gene in the very young child. *PLoS ONE* 4(11): e7845. doi: http://dx.doi.org/10.1371/journal.pone.0007845.

Suomi SJ (1997) Early determinants of behaviour: Evidence from primate studies. *Br Med Bull* 53: 170–184. doi: http://dx.doi.org/10.1093/oxfordjournals.bmb.a011598.

Susser ES, Lin SP (1992) Schizophrenia after prenatal exposure to the Dutch hunger winter of 1944–1945. *Arch Gen Psychiatry* 49: 983–988. doi: http://dx.doi.org/10.1001/archpsyc.1992.01820120071010.

Suvisaari JM, Taxell-Lassas V, Pankakoski M, Haukka JK, Lonnqvist JK, Hakkinen LT (2012) Obstetric complications as risk factors for schizophrenia spectrum psychoses in offspring of mothers with psychotic disorder. *Schizophr Bull* 39(5): 1056–1066. doi: http://dx.doi.org/10.1093/schbul/sbs109.

Tiwari AK, Zai CC, Muller DJ, Kennedy JL (2010) Genetics in schizophrenia: Where are we and what next? *Dialogues Clin Neurosci* 12(3): 289–303.

Urban N, Abi-Dargham A (2010) Neurochemical imaging in schizophrenia. *Curr Top Behav Neurosci* 4: 215–242. doi: http://dx.doi.org/10.1007/7854_2010_37.

Vaessen N, Janssen JA, Heutink P et al. (2002) Association between genetic variation in the gene for insulin-like growth factor-I and low birthweight. *Lancet* 359: 1036–1037. doi: http://dx.doi.org/10.1016/s0140-6736(02)08067-4.

van Erp TGM, Saleh PA, Rosso IM et al. (2002) Contributions of genetic risk and fetal hypoxia to hippocampal volume in patients with schizophrenia or schizoaffective disorder, their unaffected siblings, and healthy unrelated volunteers. *Am J Psychiatry* 159: 1514–1520. doi: http://dx.doi.org/10.1176/appi.ajp.159.9.1514.

van Os J, Woodruff PWR, Fananas L et al. (2000) Association between cerebral structural abnormalities and dermatoglyphic ridge counts in schizophrenia. *Compr Psychiatry* 41: 380–384. doi: http://dx.doi.org/10.1053/comp.2000.8999.

Vogeley K, Tepest R, Pfeifer U et al. (2001) Right frontal hypergyria differentiation in affected and unaffected siblings from families multiply affected with schizophrenia: A morphometric MRI study. *Am J Psychiatry* 158: 494–496. doi: http://dx.doi.org/10.1176/appi.ajp.158.3.494.

Vu TH, Chuyen NV, Li T, Hoffman AR (2003) Loss of imprinting of IGF2 sense and antisense transcripts in Wilms' tumor. *Cancer Res* 63: 1900–1905.

Wahlbeck K, Forsen T, Osmond C, Barker DJP, Eriksson JG (2001) Association of schizophrenia with low maternal body mass index, small size at birth and thinness during childhood. *Arch Gen Psychiatry* 58: 48–52. doi: http://dx.doi.org/10.1001/archpsyc.58.1.48.

Walker CK, Anderson KW, Milano KM et al. (2013) Trophoblast inclusions are significantly increased in the placentas of children in families at risk for autism. *Biol Psychiatry* 74: 204–211. doi: http://dx.doi.org/10.1016/j.biopsych.2013.03.006.

Waterland RA, Kellermayer R, Laritsky E, Rayco-Solon P, Harris RA, Travisano M et al. (2010) Season of conception in rural gambia affects DNA methylation at putative human metastable epialleles. *PLoS Genet* 6(12): e1001252. doi: http://dx.doi.org/10.1371/journal.pgen.1001252.

Wilcox AJ (2001) On the importance—and the unimportance—of birthweight. *Int J Epidemiol* 30: 1233–1241. doi: http://dx.doi.org/10.1093/ije/30.6.1233.

Wright IC, Rabe-Hesketh S, Woodruff PWR, David AS, Murray RM, Bullmore ET (2000) Meta-analysis of regional brain volumes in schizophrenia. *Am J Psychiatry* 157: 16–25. doi: http://dx.doi.org/10.1176/ajp.157.1.16.

Wright P, Takei N, Rifkin L, Murray RM (1995) Maternal influenza, obstetric complications, and schizophrenia. *Am J Psychiatry* 152: 1714–1720. doi: http://dx.doi.org/10.1176/ajp.152.12.1714.

Yang S, Platt RW, Kramer MS (2010) Variation in child cognitive ability by week of gestation among healthy term. *Am J Epidemiol* 171: 399–406. doi: http://dx.doi.org/10.1093/aje/kwp413.

11
CEREBRO-THERAPEUTICS

Philip Steer

Introduction
There are many causes of neurodisability, as outlined in previous chapters. Here, their possible prevention and amelioration are described. Although most are outside the scope of this text, that is, those of genetic (e.g. Huntingdon chorea), social (e.g. excess alcohol consumption) or environmental origin (e.g. an excess of mercury or iodine deficiency in the diet), for most, the placenta has a major role, most notably in fetal growth, preterm birth, infection and temperature control.

Prevention of fetal growth restriction
It is now well established that poor fetal growth has a lifelong impact in adulthood, including a predisposition to adult cardiovascular disease and diabetes (Godfrey et al. 2011). For many years, it was assumed that reduced nutrient transfer across the human placenta (which in severe conditions is associated with reduced oxygen transfer also) has mainly somatic effects in the fetus, with relative fetal brain growth sparing. Now with improved technologies, ultrasound imaging (and especially Doppler assessment of blood flow velocities), the changes in cerebral perfusion associated with fetal growth restriction (FGR) have been partially characterised (Hernandez-Andrade et al. 2012). With a fall in fetal cardiac output comes a relative increase in cerebral blood perfusion, this impacts upon the cerebral–placental ratio, defined by the pulsatility index of the middle cerebral and umbilical arteries. Normal values are above one, with the pulsatility index higher in the middle cerebral artery. However, as vasodilatation of blood vessels in the brain commences, and/or placental resistance increases, this ratio becomes less than one. Thus, an abnormal ratio may occur, even though individual values remain within their normal range. Vasodilatation of the cerebral vessels is thought to lead to an increased propensity for intra-cerebral and intraventricular haemorrhage. Moreover, a recent systematic review has shown that poor fetal growth (assessed as FGR or infants small for gestational age [SGA]) is associated with impaired neurodevelopmental outcomes in comparison with adequate growth (i.e. birthweight appropriate for gestational age [AGA]) (Arcangeli et al. 2012).

From these observations, it follows that prevention of FGR would be neuroprotective. On a global scale, maternal under-nutrition is an important cause of poor fetal growth and a recent meta-analysis has shown that in such populations balanced protein/energy supplementation reduces the incidence of infants being SGA by about 30% (Imdad and Bhutta 2011). In the developed world, most FGR is probably due to poor placentation, associated with maternal disorders such as pre-eclampsia and chronic hypertension; maternal nutritional interventions are therefore unlikely to be of significant benefit. Targeted nutritional interventions, such as the use of the antioxidant vitamins C and E to reduce the incidence of pre-eclampsia and FGR, have not proved beneficial (Poston et al. 2006, Rumbold et al. 2006). However, the use of therapeutic agents, such as low-dose aspirin (50–150mg daily) started before 16 weeks, gestation, has shown some value, with an approximate halving in subsequent incidence of pre-eclampsia and FGR (Bujold et al. 2009). Unfortunately, it would be inappropriate to treat the entire early pregnant population speculatively with low-dose aspirin because of complications such as gastrointestinal haemorrhage and in the meta-analysis cited, all studies for which aspirin had been started at 16 weeks or earlier included women identified to be at moderate or high risk for pre-eclampsia. Such identification is only possible in a small proportion of women, such as those with medical conditions which put them at increased risk in their first pregnancy (i.e. chronic hypertension), or the very small proportion in their second or subsequent pregnancies who have previously had the severe, early onset syndrome.

There have been many papers published in the last few years describing attempts to predict pre-eclampsia in the first trimester (e.g. using maternal serum markers or cardiovascular read-outs), but none have so far proved of sufficient sensitivity or specificity to be clinically valuable. It also remains uncertain whether low-dose aspirin would be useful in pregnancies at risk of FGR, not pre-eclampsia. Many other preventive and treatment strategies for FGR have been tried, but all have so far failed. An extensive summary of such strategies has been given by Grivell et al. (2009).

Prevention of preterm birth

Preterm birth is the leading identifiable cause of cerebral palsy (CP) (Kuban and Leviton 1994). Extreme preterm birth (before 27 weeks' gestation) is reported to result in an incidence of neurodevelopmental disability as high as 45% (Johnson et al. 2009). However, recent reports have emphasised that even late preterm births (defined as births between 34 and 37 completed weeks' gestational age) are associated with an increased rate of temperature instability, respiratory distress and clinical jaundice and a threefold increase in the need for supplemental oxygen support following birth (Loftin et al. 2010). Loftin et al. (2012, p12) point out that 'the last 6 weeks of gestation is a critical period of growth and development of the fetal brain. Brain weight at 34 weeks is only 65% of that of the term brain and gyral and sulcal formation is incomplete. Cortical volume risk of long-term neurological sequelae increases by 50% between 34 and 40 weeks' gestation and 25% of cerebellar development occurs during this period. The implication of brain immaturity in this population needs to be studied further, but there appears to be some increased susceptibility to injury that may have lasting effects'.

From the above, it follows that the prevention of preterm birth would also prevent a substantial proportion of neurodevelopmental disability. Unfortunately, spontaneous preterm birth has multiple causes: infection, spontaneous rupture of the amniotic membranes, idiopathic increases in uterine contractility, multiple pregnancy, cervical dysfunction, antepartum haemorrhage and maternal substance abuse (Steer 2005). It is clear therefore that no single therapeutic measure will be appropriate to mitigate the effect of such disparate causes. Moreover, a third of preterm births are iatrogenic, because of maternal hypertension, diabetes, antepartum haemorrhage and FGR, amongst other indications. This makes the task even more prohibitive.

Since the 1960s, tocolytics have been used in an attempt to arrest or prevent spontaneous preterm labour, ranging from alcohol through beta sympathomimetics, calcium channel blockers and oxytocin antagonists, to progesterone. Unfortunately, although many of these agents can suppress uterine contractility and even delay delivery, they have never been demonstrated to improve perinatal mortality, let alone reduce long-term disability (Ingemarsson and Lamont 2003, Dodd et al. 2008, Nassar et al. 2011, Usta et al. 2011, Abou-Ghannam et al. 2012). Indeed, in the guideline on tocolysis of women in preterm labour, published by the Royal College of Obstetricians and Gynaecologists (RCOG) in the United Kingdom (http://www.rcog.org.uk/files/rcog-corp/GTG1b26072011.pdf states that 'Use of a tocolytic drug is associated with an prolongation of pregnancy for up to 7 days but with no significant effect on preterm birth and no clear effect on perinatal or neonatal morbidity' (p3) and that 'It is reasonable not to use any tocolytic drug' (p5). It therefore seems unlikely that there will ever be a single preventative therapy for all preterm births, with an argument instead for efforts to be directed towards prevention or mitigation of the underlying pathologies.

Protective agents

STEROIDS

The use of antenatal steroids to reduce the incidence of long-term disability associated with preterm birth has been primarily directed at the prevention of respiratory distress syndrome (RDS; neonatal pulmonary surfactant deficiency). RDS causes not only hypoxia in the neonate but vascular instability, increasing the likelihood of intracerebral and intraventricular haemorrhage (Lemmers et al. 2006). It is now 40 years since Liggins and Howie published the first report of a significant reduction in the incidence of RDS in infants less than 32 weeks' gestation at birth, when mothers were treated with betamethasone for 2–7 days before delivery (Liggins and Howie 1972). During the 1980s and 1990s, the use of antenatal steroids increased greatly, accelerated by an overview of the evidence from controlled trials published in 1990 by Crowley et al. (1990). The value of a single course of steroids (usually two doses, 12 h apart) in preterm labour was further emphasised in a Cochrane review of 21 studies in 2006 (Roberts and Dalziel 2006). The authors concluded that their review supported the use of a single course of antenatal corticosteroids to reduce the incidence of not only mortality from RDS, but also neurological complications such as cerebral ventricular haemorrhage. They also concluded that there were no negative effects on the mother—in particular, no increased risk of maternal death, chorioamnionitis or puerperal sepsis.

With evidence that a single course of antenatal steroids was beneficial, many concluded that multiple courses must be better. For example, a survey by Brocklehurst et al. (1999) in the United Kingdom in 1997 showed that 98% of responding maternity units prescribed multiple courses of antenatal steroids typically for prelabour spontaneous rupture of membranes, recurrent antepartum haemorrhage, or repeated episodes of suspected preterm labour with failure to progress. This notwithstanding, concerns were expressed that multiple courses might have no additional benefit (Smith et al. 2000b) and in animal studies, they were shown to be associated with increased long-term effects, such as delayed puberty (Smith and Waddell 2000) and altered cardiovascular function (Smith et al. 2000a). These cautions were compounded with additional animal studies showing that steroids delayed myelination in the fetal brain and reduced the growth of all fetal brain areas, particularly the hippocampus (Whitelaw and Thoresen 2000).

In humans, Doyle et al. (2000) reported that antenatal corticosteroid therapy is associated with higher systolic and diastolic blood pressures in adolescence and might lead to clinical hypertension in survivors well beyond birth. Similarly, Vermillion et al. (2000) reported that multiple courses increased the risk of perinatal sepsis, without reducing the risk of intraventricular haemorrhage in the newborn infant. Subsequent reports proposed decreased neonatal head circumference (Walfisch et al. 2001), decreased birthweight (Bloom et al. 2001) and an increase in behavioural disorders, both at 3 (Newnham et al. 2002) and 6 years of age (French et al. 2004), following multiple courses of steroids. The latter study reported a statistically non-significant reduction in the incidence of CP but this may have been due to the relatively small study numbers. A protective effect against cerebral palsy was apparent, but only after controlling for confounding variables, such as intraventricular haemorrhage and periventricular leukomalacia. A further randomised trial of repeated courses of antenatal steroids compared with placebo, published in the Lancet in 2008, also showed lower birthweight, length and head circumference at birth and therefore recommended that multiple courses should not be given (Murphy et al. 2008). A follow-up at the age of 2 years, while showing that infants exposed to these multiple courses were still significantly lighter (mean weight 11.94kg, compared with 12.14kg, $p = 0.04$), reported no difference in their rates of neurlogical impairment (although unlike previous studies, the rate of cerebral palsy was not significantly higher in the multiple course group compared to placebo) (Asztalos et al. 2010). Follow-up monitoring of subsequent neuro behavioural function and school performance were advocated.

A comprehensive review in 2007 (Bonanno et al. 2007) concluded that, while there was convincing evidence that repeat courses of corticosteroids improved neonatal pulmonary outcomes and that therefore repeat treatments may be justified at very early gestations, 'enthusiasm for this treatment must be tempered by concerns about fetal growth and the lack of information on long-term safety'. The American College of Obstetrics and Gynecology (ACOG) committee opinion number 475, published in February 2011, concluded that, 'a single course of corticosteroids is recommended for pregnant women between 24 weeks and 34 weeks of gestation who are at risk of preterm delivery within 7 days' and considered that a single further 'rescue' course might be justified, but that 'repeat or multiple courses (more than two) are not recommended' (ACOG Committee on Obstetric Practice 2011).

ANTIBIOTICS

An RCOG Scientific Advisory Committee opinion paper on Intrauterine Infection and Perinatal Brain Injury (Scientific Impact Paper No 3, currently archived) in October 2007 reported that 'a growing body of epidemiological data suggests that intrauterine infection can cause brain injury in infants born before 32 weeks gestation'. Magnetic resonance imaging suggests that both white and grey matter are at risk (Inder et al. 2003), but that the major perinatal risk factors for white-matter abnormality are related to perinatal infection—'particularly maternal fever and infant sepsis'. Clinical chorioamnionitis has been linked to both periventricular leukomalacia and cerebral palsy (Wu et al. 2003). However, damage may not be primarily due to maternal infection or inflammation, but be a side effect of the fetal inflammatory response (Yoon et al. 2000). This is suggested by the elevated levels of pro-inflammatory cytokines in umbilical cord blood and amniotic fluid (notably IL-6, IL-1 beta and TNF alpha) (Yoon et al. 1996, Yoon et al. 1997). There is currently ongoing discussion in the literature about the relative importance of infection, pyrexia and inflammatory cytokines in relation to their contribution to neurodevelopmental disability. This will be considered further in the section on temperature below. However, because of the importance of infection in relation to maternal and perinatal mortality and morbidity, irrespective of long-term complications, studies of the use of antibiotics for the prevention of both preterm labour and fetal/neonatal damage have been carried out. A meta-analysis in 1996 of seven randomised clinical trials of prophylactic antibiotics in women with preterm prelabour rupture of membranes (PPROM), suggested a 50% reduction in the incidence of intraventricular haemorrhage (Egarter et al. 1996). In 2001, the Lancet published a major multicentre ORACLE I trial, testing erythromycin and co-amoxiclav (amoxicillin plus clavulanic acid) against placebo in 4826 women (Kenyon et al. 2001a). Co-amoxiclav alone or with erythromycin had no benefit over placebo with regard to the composite outcomes of neonatal death, chronic lung disease or major cerebral abnormality on ultrasonography before discharge from hospital. Nevertheless, use of erythromycin was associated with prolongation of pregnancy, reductions in neonatal treatment with surfactant, decreases in oxygen dependence at 28 or more days of age, fewer major cerebral abnormalities on ultrasonography and fewer positive blood cultures. The authors concluded that erythromycin, given to women with prelabour preterm rupture of membranes, is 'associated with a range of health benefits for the neonate and thus a probable reduction in childhood disability'. The ORACLE II trial tested the same antibiotics given to women in threatened spontaneous preterm labour and randomised 6295 women with intact membranes and without evidence of clinical infection (Kenyon et al. 2001b). In this instance, none of the trial antibiotics were associated with a lower rate of composite primary outcomes over placebo.

As a result of the ORACLE I trial, the use of erythromycin in women with prelabour preterm rupture of membranes has become ubiquitous. However, follow-up of the children born following the ORACLE I trial showed no difference between any of the groups, given antibiotics or not, in their functional impairment at 7 years of age (Kenyon et al. 2008a). Thus, the prediction of 'a probable reduction in childhood disability' was not borne out and unfortunately the follow-up of children whose mothers had been given antibiotics for threatened spontaneous preterm labour with intact membranes (the ORACLE II trial), showed the opposite effect, an impaired outcome at age of seven (Kenyon et al. 2008b) with clear functional impairments in children born to mothers prescribed with erythromycin (with or without co-amoxiclav, odds ratio 1.18, 95% CI 1.02-1.37). Most worryingly, children whose mothers had received erythromycin or co-amoxiclav more often developed cerebral palsy (erythromycin: odds ratio 1.93 (1.21–3.09); co-amoxiclav: odds ratio1.69 (1.07–2.67), giving a number needed to harm with erythromycin and co-amoxiclav of 64 and 79 patients, respectively. An editorial at the time emphasised the need for caution in giving antibiotics during pregnancy, through their potential to alter maternal gut flora and as a consequence impair the development of the naive fetal immune system (Russell and Steer 2008). Despite this warning, a subsequent study of UK practice, one year later, showed that antibiotics continued to be prescribed for spontaneous preterm labour with intact membranes in 16% of maternity units (Kenyon et al. 2010).

Of situations in which the use of antibiotics have proved less controversial, the most favourable are infants at risk of group B streptococcus infection. With recommended treatment being intravenous penicillin during labour (benzylpenicillin sodium or 'penicillin G') given as 3g (or 5 MU) intravenously at first and then 1.5g (or 2.5 MU) at 4-hourly intervals thereafter, until delivery. For women allergic to penicillin, they can be given clindamycin, 900mg intravenously every 8 hours until delivery for at least 4 hours prior to delivery (Steer and Plumb 2011).

Although over the years considerable enthusiasm has been expressed by some researchers for the use of antibiotics as a prophylactic measure to prevent preterm labour, particularly in relation to maternal bacterial vaginosis (Lamont 1999, Lamont et al. 2001), a recent review concluded that 'the current evidence suggests little benefit from routine use of antibacterials for women identified as being at risk of preterm labour' (Anonymous 2011, p.107).

MAGNESIUM SULPHATE

Magnesium sulphate infusion into the mother has been used as a tocolytic since the 1950s, especially in the United States. However, an extensive review in 2009 concluded that 'randomized clinical trials, including four comparing magnesium sulpate with placebo/control or no therapy at all, as well as 16 comparing magnesium sulfate with an alternate tocolytic regimen, failed to demonstrate its efficacy in preventing preterm birth, or reducing newborn morbidities or mortality' (Mercer and Merlino 2009, p.664). This is consistent with the conclusions described previously that no tocolytics have ever been shown to be of benefit either perinatally or longer term. Notwithstanding, this review also concluded that 'accumulating evidence indicates that magnesium sulphate treatment before anticipated early preterm birth may be protective against long-term neurologic morbidities, including cerebral palsy' (p.665). However, they cautioned against incorporating routine treatment with magnesium sulphate as a neuroprotective agent into clinical practice until further evidence had emerged, suggesting that 'if magnesium sulfate is given for neuroprotection, caregivers should follow a protocol used in one of the three major trials that have demonstrated benefits from this treatment' (Mercer and Merlino 2009, p.665).

In February 2012, a Cochrane review recounted the findings which have led to the suggestion that magnesium sulphate is neuroprotective (Bain et al. 2012). Kuban in 1992 published a study in which they investigated their previous hypothesis that pre-eclampsia reduced the risk of the infant developing germinal matrix/intraventricular haemorrhage. In addition to finding data which supported this hypothesis, they also found that administration of magnesium sulphate was associated with a reduced risk of these haemorrhages (Kuban et al. 1992). In 1995, Karin Nelson and Judith Grether carried out an observational study to investigate whether magnesium sulphate was associated with a lower prevalence of cerebral palsy. They defined an odds ratio in the exposed group of only 0.14 (95% confidence interval 0.05, 0.51) (Nelson and Grether 1995). However, they subsequently carried out a further observational study of the infants of women who did not have pre-eclampsia and found no difference in the proportion of women who had received magnesium sulphate, irrespective of their infants having cerebral palsy (Grether et al. 2000). Such inconsistency is emphasised in the 2012 Cochrane review, where five additional observational studies report protective effects for periventricular leukomalacia; one reported no beneficial effect of periventricular leukomalacia; three indicated no reduction in intraventricular haemorrhage; and five showed no reduction in cerebral palsy.

Following these contradictions, a further five prospective randomised controlled trials were conducted (Doyle et al. 2009a, 2009b). Their key finding, that antenatal magnesium sulphate treatment had no overall significant effect on fetal, neonatal or infant mortality, was consistent with its lack of efficacy as a tocolytic. However, treatment did significantly reduce the risk for cerebral palsy (overall risk ratio (RR) 0.68; 95% CI 0.54 to 0.87; five trials; 6145 infants), but this reduction was not as great as previous observational studies had maintained. While there was also a reduction in substantial gross motor dysfunction (RR 0.61; 95% CI 0.44 to 0.85; four trials; 5980 infants), there was no recorded benefit in visual, hearing or intellectual impairment. With wide variations in doses of magnesium sulphate used, the dosage at which optimal neuroprotection is conferred remains unclear. The authors therefore concluded that further studies, comparing dose, time of administration and role of maintenance therapy, were required before clear recommendations for clinical use could be proffered.

Caution regarding the premature introduction of magnesium sulphate for neuroprotection was expressed by Sibai (2011) who considered in particular, the number of women who would need to be treated if neuroprotection with magnesium sulphate became an established policy. The meta-analysis of randomised trials suggests that if magnesium sulphate was to be given to all women threatening to deliver at less than 34 weeks, the annual number of women being treated in the United States would be around 105,000. Even if only offered at gestations before 28 weeks, the number needed to be treated would still be 12,000 women. 'Despite the fact that magnesium sulphate is inexpensive and easy to give, it is associated with high rates of minor side-effects and rare but serious side-effects such as cardiorespiratory arrest and death. In addition its use requires close nursing observation and the need for enormous resources in labor and delivery' (Sibai 2011, p.297). He concluded that it was not yet appropriate to recommend its clinical use. However, in 2011 Rouse stated that 'In the United States, 2% of women deliver at <32 weeks' gestation. If these women received MgSO4 prior to delivery, > 1000 cases of handicapping cerebral palsy would be prevented safely and inexpensively every year in this country alone. To forgo this opportunity is irrationally nihilistic—it is time to use MgSO4 for fetal neuroprotection' (Rouse 2011, p. 297).

It must therefore be concluded that at the present time, there is no clear consensus about the cost/benefit of magnesium sulphate for neuroprotection. Clinicians seeking practical advice can consult guidelines from the American College of Obstetrics and Gynaecology/ the Society for Maternal Fetal Medicine (American College of Obstetricians and Gynecologists Committee on Obstetric Practice & Society for Maternal-Fetal Medicine 2010), the guidelines of the RCOG (Scientific Advisory Committee Opinion Paper 29, 2011) or the Australian Research Centre for Health of Women and Babies (2010). However, none of these documents gives a definitive recommendation.

Mode of delivery

THE PRETERM INFANT

It seems intuitive that the small, fragile preterm infant would benefit from avoiding the stress and trauma of a vaginal birth. However, Caesarean deliveries (through a poorly formed lower uterine segment or through an inadequate abdominal incision) can be equally traumatic. Between 1984 and 1986, there were three prospective randomised trials of cephalic presentations and between 1985 and 1996, three for preterm breech presentations (as summarised by Grant et al. 1996); a Cochrane update in 2009 (DOI: 10.1002/14651858. CD000078) found no subsequent studies. Notwithstanding, all six trials had problems of recruitment, because of the relative rarity of very preterm birth and the difficulty of gaining maternal consent in an emergency. The numbers randomised were 38, 4 and 2 for the cephalic presentations and 27, 38 and 13 for breech presentations. The outcomes are summarised in Table 11.1. No differences were found in the incidence of intracranial pathology,

TABLE 11.1
Maternal and neonatal outcome comparisons of Caesarean section and vaginal deliveries from six combined prospective trials of preterm cephalic and breech presentation.

Favours Caesarean section	**Odds ratio**	*p*
Maternal blood transfusion	0.02	0.03
Fetal/Infant death	0.25	0.04
Cord prolapse	0.15	0.06
Neonatal seizures	0.14	0.17
Intubation	0.58	0.19
Low 5 min Apgar	0.61	0.3
Favours vaginal birth		
Low cord pH	10.8	0.01
Major maternal complications	6.4	0.01
Breastfeeding	20.0	0.16
Postpartum hemorrhage	9.5	0.3
Need for mechanical ventilation	2.12	0.5
Head entrapment	4.5	0.5

alterative birth trauma, neonatal stay in hospital (exceeding 10 days), maternal stay (exceeding 10 days), or abnormal follow-up in childhood. The overall conclusion was that Caesarean section may have some benefits for the infants, but this has to be weighed against the increased risk to the mother, which is often difficult in situations of a poorly formed lower uterine segment.

TERM BREECH PRESENTATION

There have been three prospective randomised trials of elective Caesarean section in the fetus in breech presentation, the meta-analysis of which is dominated by the Canadian term breech trial (Hannah et al. 2000). There can now be little doubt from these studies (and confirmed by observational studies which have followed) that perinatal mortality is significantly and substantially reduced (at least in developed countries) by elective Caesarean section [risk ratio 0.33 (95% CI 0.19, 0.56)]. However, there was no reduction in subsequent deaths or neurodevelopmental delay, at least at two years of age (RR 1.09: 0.52, 2.30) (Hofmeyr et al. 2011).

TERM CEPHALIC PRESENTATION

A large study of newborn encephalopathy in term infants was carried out as part of the Western Australian case-control study between June 1993 and September 1995. This study suggested a protective effect of elective Caesarean section (before the onset of labour), with rates of 14.5% in the control group and 3.7% in pregnancies where the infant had newborn encephalopathy (Badawi et al. 1998). Nevertheless, the suggestion that elective Caesarean section for uncomplicated pregnancies with cephalic presentation might be protective is highly controversial, as there are currently no published results of randomised trials of mode of delivery for the term cephalic infant.

CONTINUOUS ELECTRONIC INTRAPARTUM FETAL MONITORING AND CAESAREAN SECTION

While there is continuing controversy about the proportion of neurodevelopmental disability attributed to intrapartum events, there can be no doubt that at least some instances of spastic cerebral palsy are due to birth asphyxia. Birth asphyxia is defined as (1) an umbilical artery pH less than seven, (2) a five-minute Apgar score less than or equal to 3, (3) moderate or severe neonatal encephalopathy and (4) multi-organ dysfunction (ACOG 1991). The introduction of continuous electronic fetal heart rate monitoring in the 1960s was aimed at detecting hypoxic changes in the fetal heart rate pattern, allowing prompt delivery before brain damage had occurred. Initially it was greeted with great enthusiasm (Beard et al. 1977), but its association with a rising Caesarean section rate prompted a number of prospective randomised controlled trials. A meta-analysis of nine such trials in 1995 by Vintzileos et al, confirmed a significant rise in Caesarean sections associated with its use (from 3.8 to 5.2%), but the associated fall in perinatal mortality from 4.9 to 4.2 per thousand was not statistically significant (Vintzileos et al. 1995). However, when the perinatal deaths were classified by cause, the odds ratio of hypoxic death was 0.41 (0.7 per thousand compared with 1.8 per thousand). Further, a meta-analysis including three additional trials published in the same year by Thacker et al. (2001), reported a statistically significant 50% reduction in neonatal seizures associated with the use of routine electronic fetal monitoring. The controversy has continued, but most clinicians continue to use the technique. More recently, Dyson et al. summarised the evidence that continuous fetal heart rate monitoring in labour, can benefit long-term neurodevelopment of the infant, by reducing the incidence of neonatal seizures (Dyson et al. 2011).

The use of computer aided fetal heart rate pattern interpretation is currently being studied in a prospective randomised controlled trial of 46,000 labours (the INFANT STUDY, https://www.npeu.ox.ac.uk/infant). This study includes an assessment of neurodevelopment in 7000 infants at 2 years of age.

TEMPERATURE CONTROL

As mentioned previously, there is thought to be a significant link between antenatal and intrapartum infection and damage to the fetal brain, resulting in permanent disability. In 1997, Grether et al. reported that maternal fever exceeding 38°C in labour was associated with an increased risk of unexplained cerebral palsy (OR 9.3; 95%, CI 2.7-31.0), as was clinical diagnosis of chorioamnionitis. The assumption was made that fever in labour indicated an infectious process, apparently confirmed by a report in the subsequent year from the Western Australian case-control study, showing maternal pyrexia as a risk factor for newborn encephalopathy (OR 3.82) (Badawi et al. 1998). However, this assumption was questioned and foreshadowed by the publication in 1989 of a study linking the use of regional analgesia (epidural anaesthesia) with a rise in maternal temperature (Fusi et al. 1989), an observation subsequently confirmed by many others (Camann et al., et al. 1993, Mercier and Benhamou 1994, Herbst et al. 1995, Mayer et al. 1997).

In 1997, Lieberman et al. published data strongly suggesting that many cases of intrapartum pyrexia assumed to be due to infection were in fact the result of epidural anaesthesia (Lieberman et al. 1997). They studied 1657 nulliparous women with term pregnancies and singleton vertex fetuses who were afebrile at admission for delivery. Without epidural the rate of fever remained low, regardless of length of labour; but with epidural anaesthesia fever increased from 7% for labours up to 6 hours, to 36% for labours greater than 18 hours. Neonates whose mothers received epidurals were more often evaluated for sepsis (34.0% vs 9.8%; adjusted OR 5 4.3, 95% CI 5 3.2, 5.9) and treated with antibiotics (15.4% vs 3.8%; adjusted OR 5 3.9, 95% CI 5 2.1, 6.1). To clarify their observations, Lieberman et al. subsequently studied neonatal outcomes for 1218 nulliparous women in spontaneous labour without signs of infection other than fever (Lieberman et al. 2000). Of these, 123 had a fever greater than 38°C (120 had epidurals) and 23% had infants with a one-minute Apgar score of less than 7, compared to only 8% without fever. Of infants whose mothers experienced fever, 3.3% had seizures, compared to only 0.2% apyrexic mothers. This group since published a further study, in which the incidence of pyrexia greater than 38°C was 19.2% in women receiving epidural anaesthesia compared with 2.4% for those who did not (Greenwell et al. 2012). Amongst women receiving an epidural, a significant linear trend was observed between maximum maternal temperature and all adverse neonatal outcomes examined, including hypotonia, assisted ventilation, 1- and 5-min Apgar scores less than 7 and early-onset seizures.

A further link between intrapartum fever and encephalopathy has also been reported by Impey et al. (2001) who found a crude odds ratio of 10.8, a relationship which persisted after adjustment for covariates. This group have also reported an interaction between intra-partum fever and fetal acidosis. When the infants were born acidotic, there was an adjusted odds ratio of 11.5 for encephalopathy and this increased to 93.9 if the mother had also been pyrexial (Impey et al. 2008).

In essence, pyrexia increases tissue metabolic rate and therefore oxygen requirements. However, Castillo et al. (1999) have suggested that the rise in temperature also produces an increase in neurotoxic oxygen free radicals and glutamate. Animal studies have sup-ported an interaction between ischaemia and hyperthermia. For example, hyperthermia worsens the effect of brain ischaemia in dogs (Wass et al. 1995) and may increase damage in human stroke (Hajat et al. 2000). Preventing temperature rise has shown protection in the rat brain against ischaemic effects (Li et al. 1999).

Many substantial studies and randomised controlled trials over the last decade have established neonatal head cooling as protection against the effects of hypoxia (Sirimanne et al. 1996, Gunn et al. 1998, Gluckman et al. 2005, Shankaran et al. 2005, Azzopardi et al. 2008, 2009, Battin et al. 2001, Edwards et al. 2010). Gunn and Bennet have suggested that 'there are now strong case control data to suggest that even mild pyrexia during labour has an adverse impact on fetuses exposed to hypoxia ischaemia, increasing the risk of subsequent encephalopathy. Thus, when maternal pyrexia develops, as well as appropriate screening and treatment for infection, lowering the maternal fever should be the desired goal' (Gunn and Bennet 2001, p. 246). Under these circumstances the fetus may be particularly at risk, because in order to dissipate the heat generated by its metabolism down a temperature gradient, its core temperature has to be approximately 0.9°C above that of the mother (Gurney Champion 1903, Wood and Beard 1964, Macaulay et al. 1992a, Macaulay et al. 1992b).

The mechanism by which epidural anaesthesia provokes maternal pyrexia remains con-troversial. Our own group has been investigating the hypothesis that heat loss is reduced by the blocking of the autonomic outflow to the lower limbs, thus preventing sweating and by reducing maternal hyperventilation. We also suggest that the thermal control centre in the hypothalamus is disturbed by the blockage of temperature signals from the lower half of the body (the axons of temperature neurons are of similar diameter to those of pain neurons and are thus blocked by similar concentrations of local anaesthetic), producing an impression that the body is too cold (Banerjee and Steer 2003). Preliminary trials of a neck warmer to increase the temperature of the blood perfusing the hypothalamus, thereby resetting body temperature control to a lower level, are promising. However, an alternative hypothesis is that the pyrexia produced by epidurals is secondary to inflammatory changes. This is sup-ported by evidence of high initial levels (Unal et al. 2011) and rises of interleukin-6 (Riley et al. 2011) induced by epidural anaesthesia. It has also been suggested that increased oxida-tive stress at the beginning of labour contributes to the development of pyrexia (Goetzl et al. 2010). This suggestion, that the process is inflammatory rather than infectious, is supported by the lack of evidence of any increased rate of infection on placental histology associated with the use of epidurals (Riley et al. 2011). A randomised study of the use of intravenous methylprednisolone showed that very high doses (100mg, four hourly) prevented an increase in maternal fever following the use of epidural anaesthesia, although smaller doses (25mg, eight hourly) had no effect (Goetzl et al. 2006). Regardless, the use of such high doses would be likely to have unwanted side effects and a more recent small trial of epidural (rather than systemic) dexamethasone has shown promise (Wang et al. 2011). A recent review by Segal (2010, p.1467) concluded that 'maternal inflammatory fever is associated with neonatal brain injury, manifest as cerebral palsy, encephalopathy and learning deficits in later childhood. At present, there are no safe and effective means to inhibit epidural-associated fever. Future research should define the aetiology of this fever and search for safe and effective interventions to prevent it and to inhibit its potential adverse effects on the neonatal brain.'

REFERENCES

Abou-Ghannam G, Usta IM, Nassar AH (2012) Indomethacin in pregnancy: Applications and safety. *Am J Perinatol* 29(3): 175–186. doi: http://dx.doi.org/10.1055/s-0031-1284227

ACOG (1991) Utility of umbilical cord blood acid-base measurement: ACOG Committee Opinion. *Obstet Gynecol* 91: 33–34.

ACOG committee on Obstetric Practice (2011) ACOG Committee Opinion No. 475: Antenatal corticosteroid therapy for fetal maturation. *Obstet Gynecol* 117: 422–424. doi: http://dx.doi.org/10.1097/aog.0b013e31820eee00

American College of Obstetricians and Gynecologists Committee on Obstetric Practice and Society for Maternal-Fetal Medicine (2010) Committee Opinion No. 455: Magnesium sulfate before anticipated preterm birth for neuroprotection. *Obstet Gynecol* 115: 669–671. doi: http://dx.doi.org/10.1097/aog.0b013e3181d4ffa5

Anonymous (2011) The role of antibacterials in women at risk of preterm birth. *Drug Ther Bull* 49(9): 105–108. doi: http://dx.doi.org/10.1136/dtb.2011.02.0056

Arcangeli T, Thilaganathan B, Hooper R, Khan KS, Bhide A (2012) Neurodevelopmental delay in small babies at term. A systematic review. *Ultrasound Obstet Gynecol* 40(3): 267–275. doi: http://dx.doi.org/10.1002/uog.11112

Asztalos EV, Murphy KE, Hannah ME et al. (2010) Multiple courses of antenatal corticosteroids for preterm birth study: 2-year outcomes. *Pediatrics* 126(5): e1045–e1055. doi: http://dx.doi.org/10.1542/peds.2010-0857

Australian Research Centre for Health of Women and Babies (2010) Antenatal Magnesium Sulphate Prior to Preterm Birth for Neuroprotection of the Fetus, Infant and Child – National Clinical Practice Guidelines. [online]. Available http://www.adelaide.edu.au/arch/MagnesiumSulphate2010.pdf.

Azzopardi D, Brocklehurst P, Edwards D et al. (2008) The TOBY study. Whole body hypothermia for the treatment of perinatal asphyxial encephalopathy: A randomised controlled trial. *BMC Pediatr* 8(17): 17. doi: http://dx.doi.org/10.1186/1471-2431-8-17

Azzopardi DV, Strohm B, Edwards AD et al. (2009) Moderate hypothermia to treat perinatal asphyxial encephalopathy. *N Engl J Med* 361(14): 1349–1358. doi: http://dx.doi.org/10.1056/nejmoa0900854

Badawi N, Kurinczuk JJ, Keogh JM et al. (1998) Intrapartum risk factors for newborn encephalopathy: The Western Australian case-control study. *BMJ* 317(7172): 1554–1558. doi: http://dx.doi.org/10.1136/bmj.317.7172.1554

Bain E, Middleton P, Crowther CA (2012) Different magnesium sulphate regimens for neuroprotection of the fetus for women at risk of preterm birth. *Cochrane Database Syst Rev* 2: CD009302. doi: http://dx.doi.org/10.1002/14651858.CD009302.pub2

Banerjee S, Steer PJ (2003) The rise in maternal temperature associated with epidural analgesia is harmful and should be treated. *Int J Obstet Anaesth* 12: 280–286.

Battin MR, Dezoete JA, Gunn TR, Gluckman PD, Gunn AJ (2001) Neurodevelopmental outcome of infants treated with head cooling and mild hypothermia after perinatal asphyxia. *Pediatrics* 107(3): 480–484. doi: http://dx.doi.org/10.1542/peds.107.3.480

Beard RW, Edington PT, Sibanda J (1977) The effects of routine intrapartum monitoring on clinical practice. *Contrib Gynecol Obstet* 3(14–21): 14–21.

Bloom SL, Sheffield JS, McIntire DD, Leveno KJ (2001) Antenatal dexamethasone and decreased birth weight. *Obstet Gynecol* 97(4): 485–490. doi: http://dx.doi.org/10.1016/s0029-7844(00)01206-0

Bonanno C, Fuchs K, Wapner RJ (2007) Single versus repeat courses of antenatal steroids to improve neonatal outcomes: Risks and benefits. *Obstet Gynecol Surv* 62(4): 261–271. doi: http://dx.doi.org/10.1097/01.ogx.0000259226.62431.78

Brocklehurst P, Gates S, McKenzie-McHarg K, Alfirevic Z, Chamberlain G (1999) Are we prescribing multiple courses of antenatal corticosteroids? A survey of practice in the UK. *Br J Obstet Gynecol* 106(9): 977–979. doi: http://dx.doi.org/10.1111/j.1471-0528.1999.tb08440.x

Bujold E, Morency AM, Roberge S, Lacasse Y, Forest JC, Giguere Y (2009) Acetylsalicylic acid for the prevention of preeclampsia and intra-uterine growth restriction in women with abnormal uterine artery Doppler: A systematic review and meta-analysis. *J Obstet Gynecol Can* 31(9): 818–826.

Camann WR, Hortvet LA, Hughes N, Bader AM, Datta S (1991) Maternal temperature regulation during extradural analgesia for labour. *Br J Anaesth* 67(5): 565–568. doi: http://dx.doi.org/10.1093/bja/67.5.565

Castillo J, Davalos A, Noya M (1999) Aggravation of acute ischemic stroke by hyperthermia is related to an excitotoxic mechanism. *Cerebrovasc Dis* 9(1): 22–27. doi: http://dx.doi.org/10.1159/000015891

Crowley P, Chalmers I, Keirse MJ (1990) The effects of corticosteroid administration before preterm delivery: An overview of the evidence from controlled trials. *Br J Obstet Gynecol* 97(1): 11–25. doi: http://dx.doi.org/10.1111/j.1471-0528.1990.tb01711.x

Dodd JM, Flenady VJ, Cincotta R, Crowther CA (2008) Progesterone for the prevention of preterm birth: A systematic review. *Obstet Gynecol* 112(1): 127–134. doi: http://dx.doi.org/10.1097/AOG.0b013e31817d0262

Doyle LW, Crowther CA, Middleton P, Marret S (2009a) Antenatal magnesium sulfate and neurologic outcome in preterm infants: A systematic review. *Obstet Gynecol* 113(6): 1327–1333. doi: http://dx.doi.org/10.1097/aog.0b013e3181a60495

Doyle LW, Crowther CA, Middleton P, Marret S, Rouse D (2009b) Magnesium sulphate for women at risk of preterm birth for neuroprotection of the fetus. *Cochrane Database Syst Rev* (1): CD004661.

Doyle LW, Ford GW, Davis NM., Callanan C (2000) Antenatal corticosteroid therapy and blood pressure at 14 years of age in preterm children. *Clin Sci* (Lond) 98(2): 137–142.

Dyson C, Austin T, Lees C (2011) Could routine cardiotocography reduce long term cognitive impairment? *BMJ* 342: d3120. doi: http://dx.doi.org/10.1136/bmj.d3120

Edwards AD, Brocklehurst P, Gunn AJ et al. (2010) Neurological outcomes at 18 months of age after moderate hypothermia for perinatal hypoxic ischaemic encephalopathy: Synthesis and meta-analysis of trial data. *BMJ* 340: c363. doi: http://dx.doi.org/10.1136/bmj.c363

Egarter C, Leitich H, Karas H et al. (1996) Antibiotic treatment in preterm premature rupture of membranes and neonatal morbidity: A metaanalysis [see comments]. *Am J Obstet Gynecol* 174(2): 589–597. doi: http://dx.doi.org/10.1016/s0002-9378(96)70433-7

French NP, Hagan R, Evans SF, Mullan A, Newnham JP (2004) Repeated antenatal corticosteroids: Effects on cerebral palsy and childhood behavior. *Am J Obstet Gynecol* 190(3): 588–595. doi: http://dx.doi.org/10.1016/j.ajog.2003.12.016

Fusi L, Steer PJ, Maresh MJA, Beard RW (1989) Maternal pyrexia associated with the use of epidural anaesthesia in labour. *Lancet* i: 1250–1252. doi: http://dx.doi.org/10.1016/S0140-6736(89)92341-6

Gluckman PD, Wyatt JS, Azzopardi D et al. (2005) Selective head cooling with mild systemic hypothermia after neonatal encephalopathy: Multicentre randomised trial. *Lancet* 365(9460): 663–670. doi: http://dx.doi.org/10.1016/s0140-6736(05)17946-x

Godfrey KM, Inskip HM, Hanson MA (2011) The long-term effects of prenatal development on growth and metabolism. *Semin Reprod Med* 29(3): 257–265. doi: http://dx.doi.org/10.1055/s-0031-1275518

Goetzl L, Manevich Y, Roedner C, Praktish A, Hebbar L, Townsend DM (2010) Maternal and fetal oxidative stress and intrapartum term fever. *Am J Obstet Gynecol* 202(4): 363–365. doi: http://dx.doi.org/10.1016/j.ajog.2010.01.034

Goetzl L, Zighelboim I, Badell M et al. (2006) Maternal corticosteroids to prevent intrauterine exposure to hyperthermia and inflammation: A randomized, double-blind, placebo-controlled trial. *Am J Obstet Gynecol* 195(4): 1031–1037. doi: http://dx.doi.org/10.1016/j.ajog.2006.06.012

Grant A, Penn ZJ, Steer PJ (1996) Elective or selective Caesarean delivery of the small baby? A systematic review of the controlled trials. *Br J Obstet Gynecol* 103: 1197–1200. doi: http://dx.doi.org/10.1111/j.1471-0528.1996.tb09628.x

Greenwell EA, Wyshak G, Ringer SA, Johnson LC, Rivkin MJ, Lieberman E (2012) Intrapartum temperature elevation, epidural use, and adverse outcome in term infants. *Pediatrics* 129(2): e447–e454. doi: 10.1542/peds.2010-2301. Epub 2012 Jan 30.

Grether JK, Hoogstrate J, Walsh-Greene E, Nelson KB (2000) Magnesium sulfate for tocolysis and risk of spastic cerebral palsy in premature children born to women without preeclampsia. *Am J Obstet Gynecol* 183(3): 717–725. doi: http://dx.doi.org/10.1067/mob.2000.106581

Grether JK, Nelson KB (1997) Maternal infection and cerebral palsy in infants of normal birth weight. *JAMA* 278(3): 207–211. doi: http://dx.doi.org/10.1001/jama.1997.03550030047032

Grivell R, Dodd J, Robinson J (2009) The prevention and treatment of intrauterine growth restriction. *Best Pract Res Clin Obstet Gynecol* 23(6): 795–807. doi: http://dx.doi.org/10.1016/j.bpobgyn.2009.06.004

Gunn AJ, Bennet L (2001) Is temperature important in delivery room resuscitation? *Semin Neonatol* 6(3): 241–249. doi: http://dx.doi.org/10.1053/siny.2001.0052

Gunn AJ, Gunn TR, Gunning MI, Williams CE, Gluckman PD (1998) Neuroprotection with prolonged head cooling started before postischemic seizures in fetal sheep. *Pediatrics* 102(5): 1098–1106.

Gurney Champion S (1903) Observations of the relationship of the maternal and foetal temperatures. *J Obstet Gynecol Br Emp* 3: 556–557. doi: http://dx.doi.org/10.1111/j.1471-0528.1903.tb06928.x

Hajat C, Hajat S, Sharma P (2000) Effects of poststroke pyrexia on stroke outcome: A meta-analysis of studies in patients. *Stroke* 31(2): 410–414. doi: http://dx.doi.org/10.1161/01.str.31.2.410

Hannah ME, Hannah WJ, Hewson SA, Hodnett ED, Saigal S, Willan AR (2000) Planned Caesarean section versus planned vaginal birth for breech presentation at term: A randomised multicentre trial. Term Breech Trial Collaborative Group. *Lancet* 356(9239): 1375–1383. doi: http://dx.doi.org/10.1016/s0140-6736(00)02840-3

Herbst A, Wolner-Hanssen P, Ingemarsson I (1995) Risk factors for fever in labor. *Obstet Gynecol* 86(5): 790–794. doi: http://dx.doi.org/10.1016/0029-7844(95)00254-o

Hernandez-Andrade E, Benavides Serralde JA, Cruz-Martinez R (2012) Can anomalies of fetal brain circulation be useful in the management of growth restricted fetuses? *Prenat Diagn* 32(2): 103–112. doi: 10.1002/pd.2913 [doi].

Hofmeyr GJ, Hannah M, Lawrie A (2011) Planned Caesarean section for term breech delivery. [online]. Available http://onlinelibrary.wiley.com/doi/10.1002/14651858.CD000166/full.

Imdad A, Bhutta ZA (2011) Effect of balanced protein energy supplementation during pregnancy on birth outcomes. *BMC Public Health* 11(Suppl 3): S17. doi: http://dx.doi.org/10.1186/1471-2458-11-s3-s17

Impey L, Greenwood C, MacQuillan K, Reynolds M, Sheil O (2001) Fever in labour and neonatal encephalopathy: A prospective cohort study. *Br J Obstet Gynecol* 108(6): 594–597. doi: http://dx.doi.org/10.1016/s0306-5456(00)00145-5

Impey LW, Greenwood CE, Black RS, Yeh PS, Sheil O, Doyle P (2008) The relationship between intrapartum maternal fever and neonatal acidosis as risk factors for neonatal encephalopathy. *Am J Obstet Gynecol* 198(1): 49–46. doi: http://dx.doi.org/10.1016/j.ajog.2007.06.011

Inder TE, Wells SJ, Mogridge NB, Spencer C, Volpe JJ (2003) Defining the nature of the cerebral abnormalities in the premature infant: A qualitative magnetic resonance imaging study. *J Pediatr* 143(2): 171–179. doi: http://dx.doi.org/10.1067/s0022-3476(03)00357-3

Ingemarsson I, Lamont RF (2003) An update on the controversies of tocolytic therapy for the prevention of preterm birth. *Acta Obstet Gynecol Scand* 82(1): 1–9. doi: http://dx.doi.org/10.1080/j.1600-0412.2003.820101.x

Johnson S, Hennessy EM, Smith R, Trikic R, Wolke D, Marlow N (2009) Academic attainment and special educational needs in extremely preterm children at 11 years of age: The EPICure study. *Arch Dis Child* 94(4): F283–F289. doi: http://dx.doi.org/10.1136/adc.2008.152793

Kenyon S, Pike K, Jones D et al. (2010) Has publication of the results of the ORACLE Children Study changed practice in the UK? *BJOG* 117(11): 1344–1349. doi: http://dx.doi.org/10.1111/j.1471-0528.2010.02661.x

Kenyon S, Pike K, Jones DR et al. (2008a) Childhood outcomes after prescription of antibiotics to pregnant women with preterm rupture of the membranes: 7-year follow-up of the ORACLE I trial. *Lancet* 372(9646): 1310–1318. doi: http://dx.doi.org/10.1016/s0140-6736(08)61202-7

Kenyon S, Pike K, Jones DR et al. (2008b) Childhood outcomes after prescription of antibiotics to pregnant women with spontaneous preterm labour: 7-year follow-up of the ORACLE II trial. *Lancet* 372(9646): 1319–1327. doi: http://dx.doi.org/10.1016/s0140-6736(08)61203-9

Kenyon SL, Taylor DJ, Tarnow-Mordi W (2001a) Broad-spectrum antibiotics for preterm, prelabour rupture of fetal membranes: The ORACLE I randomised trial. ORACLE Collaborative Group. *Lancet* 357(9261): 979–988. doi: http://dx.doi.org/10.1016/s0140-6736(00)04233-1

Kenyon SL, Taylor DJ, Tarnow-Mordi W (2001b) Broad-spectrum antibiotics for spontaneous preterm labour: The ORACLE II randomised trial. ORACLE Collaborative Group. *Lancet* 357(9261): 989–994. doi: http://dx.doi.org/10.1016/s0140-6736(00)04234-3

Kuban KC, Leviton A (1994) Cerebral palsy. *N Engl J Med* 330(3): 188–195.

Kuban KC, Leviton A, Pagano M, Fenton T, Strassfeld R, Wolff M (1992) Maternal toxemia is associated with reduced incidence of germinal matrix hemorrhage in premature babies. *J Child Neurol* 7(1): 70–76. doi: http://dx.doi.org/10.1177/088307389200700113

Lamont RF (1999) The prevention of preterm birth with the use of antibiotics. *Eur J Pediatr* 158(Suppl 1): S2–S4. doi: http://dx.doi.org/10.1007/pl00014313

Lamont RF, Taylor-Robinson D, Hay PE (2001) Antibiotics for adverse outcomes of pregnancy. *Lancet* 358(9294): 1728–1729. doi: http://dx.doi.org/10.1016/s0140-6736(01)06748-4

Lemmers PM, Toet M, van Schelven LJ, van Bel F 2006. Cerebral oxygenation and cerebral oxygen extraction in the preterm infant: The impact of respiratory distress syndrome. *Exp Brain Res* 173(3): 458–467. doi: http://dx.doi.org/10.1007/s00221-006-0388-8

Li F, Omae T, Fisher M (1999) Spontaneous hyperthermia and its mechanism in the intraluminal suture middle cerebral artery occlusion model of rats. *Stroke* 30(11): 2464–2470.

Lieberman E, Lang JM, Frigoletto F Jr, Richardson DK, Ringer SA, Cohen A (1997) Epidural analgesia, intrapartum fever, and neonatal sepsis evaluation. *Pediatrics* 99(3): 415–419. doi: http://dx.doi.org/10.1542/peds.99.3.415

Lieberman E, Lang J, Richardson DK, Frigoletto FD, Heffner LJ, Cohen A (2000) Intrapartum maternal fever and neonatal outcome. *Pediatrics* 105(1 Pt 1): 8–13.

Liggins GC, Howie RN (1972) A controlled trial of antepartum glucocorticoid treatment for prevention of the respiratory distress syndrome in premature infants. *Pediatrics* 50(4): 515–525.

Loftin RW, Habli M, Snyder CC, Cormier CM, Lewis DF, Defranco EA (2010) Late preterm birth. *Rev Obstet Gynecol* 3(1): 10–19.

Macaulay JH, Bond K, Steer PJ (1992a) Epidural analgesia in labor and fetal hyperthermia. *Obstet Gynecol* 80: 665–669.

Macaulay JH, Randall NR, Bond K, Steer PJ (1992b). Continuous monitoring of fetal temperature by noninvasive probe and its relationship to maternal temperature, fetal heart rate, and cord arterial oxygen and pH. *Obstet Gynecol* 79: 469–474. doi: http://dx.doi.org/10.1097/00006250-199203000-00029

Mayer DC, Chescheir NC, Spielman FJ (1997) Increased intrapartum antibiotic administration associated with epidural analgesia in labor. *Am J Perinatol* 14(2): 83–86. doi: http://dx.doi.org/10.1055/s-2007-994103

Mercer BM, Merlino AA (2009) Magnesium sulfate for preterm labor and preterm birth. *Obstet Gynecol* 114(3): 650–668. doi: http://dx.doi.org/10.1097/aog.0b013e3181b48336

Mercier FJ, Benhamou D (1994) Hyperthermia after obstetrical epidural anesthesia [French]. *Cahiers d Anesthesiologie* 42(2): 257–260.

Murphy KE, Hannah ME, Willan AR et al. (2008) Multiple courses of antenatal corticosteroids for preterm birth (MACS): A randomised controlled trial. *Lancet* 372(9656): 2143–2151. doi: http://dx.doi.org/10.1016/s0140-6736(08)61929-7

Nassar AH, Aoun J, Usta IM (2011) Calcium channel blockers for the management of preterm birth: A review. *Am J Perinatol* 28(1): 57–66. doi: http://dx.doi.org/10.1055/s-0030-1262512

Nelson KB, Grether JK (1995) Can magnesium sulfate reduce the risk of cerebral palsy in very low birth weight infants? *Pediatrics* 95(2): 263–269.

Newnham JP, Moss TJ, Nitsos I, Sloboda DM (2002) Antenatal corticosteroids: The good, the bad and the unknown. *Curr Opin Obstet Gynecol* 14(6): 607–612. doi: http://dx.doi.org/10.1097/00001703-200212000-00006

Poston L, Briley AL, Seed PT, Kelly FJ, Shennan AH (2006) Vitamin C and vitamin E in pregnant women at risk for pre-eclampsia (VIP trial): Randomised placebo-controlled trial. *Lancet* 367(9517): 1145–1154. doi: http://dx.doi.org/10.1016/s0140-6736(06)68433-x

Riley LE, Celi AC, Onderdonk AB et al. (2011) Association of epidural-related fever and noninfectious inflammation in term labor. *Obstet Gynecol* 117(3): 588–595. doi: http://dx.doi.org/10.1097/aog.0b013e31820b0503

Roberts D, Dalziel S (2006) Antenatal corticosteroids for accelerating fetal lung maturation for women at risk of preterm birth. *Cochrane Database Syst Rev* (3): CD004454. doi: http://dx.doi.org/10.1002/14651858.CD004454.pub2

Rouse DJ (2011) Magnesium sulfate for fetal neuroprotection. *Am J Obstet Gynecol* 205(4): 296–297. doi: http://dx.doi.org/10.1016/j.ajog.2011.02.083

Rumbold AR, Crowther CA, Haslam RR et al. (2006) Vitamins C and E and the risks of preeclampsia and perinatal complications. *N Engl J Med* 354(17): 1796–1806. doi: http://dx.doi.org/10.1056/nejmoa054186

Russell AR, Steer PJ (2008) Antibiotics in preterm labour--the ORACLE speaks. *Lancet* 372(9646): 1276–1278. doi: http://dx.doi.org/10.1016/s0140-6736(08)61248-9

Scientific Advisory Committee Opinion Paper 29 (2011) Magnesium sulphate to prevent cerebral palsy following pretermbirth. [online]. Available http://www.rcog.org.uk/files/rcog-corp/28.9.11SACMagnesium.pdf.

Segal S (2010) Labor epidural analgesia and maternal fever. *Anesth Analg* 111(6): 1467–1475. doi: http://dx.doi.org/10.1213/ane.0b013e3181f713d4

Shankaran S, Laptook AR, Ehrenkranz RA et al. (2005) Whole-body hypothermia for neonates with hypoxic-ischemic encephalopathy. *N Engl J Med* 353(15): 1574–1584. doi: http://dx.doi.org/10.1056/nejmcps050929

Sibai BM (2011) Magnesium sulfate for neuroprotection in patients at risk for early preterm delivery: Not yet. *Am J Obstet Gynecol* 205(4): 296–297. doi: http://dx.doi.org/10.1016/j.ajog.2011.02.084

Sirimanne ES, Blumberg RM, Bossano D et al. 1996. The effect of prolonged modification of cerebral temperature on outcome after hypoxic-ischemic brain injury in the infant rat. *Pediatr Res* 39(4 Pt 1): 591–597. doi: http://dx.doi.org/10.1203/00006450-199604000-00005

Smith JT, Waddell BJ (2000) Increased fetal glucocorticoid exposure delays puberty onset in postnatal life. *Endocrinology* 141(7): 2422–2428. doi: http://dx.doi.org/10.1210/endo.141.7.7541

Smith LM, Ervin MG, Wada N, Ikegami M, Polk DH, Jobe AH (2000a) Antenatal glucocorticoids alter postnatal preterm lamb renal and cardiovascular responses to intravascular volume expansion. *Pediatr Res* 47(5): 622–627. doi: http://dx.doi.org/10.1203/00006450-200005000-00011

Smith LM, Qureshi N, Chao CR (2000b) Effects of single and multiple courses of antenatal glucocorticoids in preterm newborns less than 30 weeks' gestation. *J Matern Fetal Med* 9(2): 131–135. doi: http://dx.doi.org/10.3109/14767050009053438

Steer P (2005) The epidemiology of preterm labor—a global perspective. *J Perinat Med* 33(4): 273–276. doi: http://dx.doi.org/10.1515/jpm.2005.053

Steer PJ, Plumb J (2011) Myth: Group B streptococcal infection in pregnancy: Comprehended and conquered. *Semin Fetal Neonatal Med* 16(5): 254–258. doi: http://dx.doi.org/10.1016/j.siny.2011.03.005

Thacker SB, Stroup D, Chang M (2001) Continuous electronic heart rate monitoring for fetal assessment during labor. Cochrane Database Syst Rev (2): CD000063. doi: http://dx.doi.org/10.1002/14651858.CD000063.

Unal ER, Cierny JT, Roedner C, Newman R, Goetzl L (2011) Maternal inflammation in spontaneous term labor. *Am J Obstet Gynecol* 204(3): 223–225. doi: http://dx.doi.org/10.1016/j.ajog.2011.01.002

Usta IM, Khalil A, Nassar AH (2011) Oxytocin antagonists for the management of preterm birth: A review. *Am J Perinatol* 28(6): 449–460. doi: http://dx.doi.org/10.1055/s-0030-1270111

Vermillion ST, Soper DE, Newman RB (2000) Neonatal sepsis and death after multiple courses of antenatal betamethasone therapy. *Am J Obstet Gynecol* 183(4): 810–814. doi: http://dx.doi.org/10.1067/mob.2000.108838

Vinson DC, Thomas R, Kiser T (1993) Association between epidural analgesia during labor and fever. *J Fam Pract* 36(6): 617–622.

Vintzileos AM, Nochimson DJ, Guzman ER, Knuppel RA, Lake M, Schifrin BS (1995) Intrapartum electronic fetal heart rate monitoring versus intermittent auscultation: A meta-analysis. *Obstet Gynecol* 85(1): 149–155. doi: http://dx.doi.org/10.1016/0029-7844(94)00320-d

Walfisch A, Hallak M, Mazor M (2001) Multiple courses of antenatal steroids: Risks and benefits. *Obstet Gynecol* 98(3): 491–497. doi: http://dx.doi.org/10.1016/s0029-7844(01)01368-0

Wang LZ, Hu XX, Liu X, Qian P, Ge JM, Tang BL (2011) Influence of epidural dexamethasone on maternal temperature and serum cytokine concentration after labor epidural analgesia. *Int J Gynecol Obstet* 113(1): 40–43. doi: http://dx.doi.org/10.1016/j.ijgo.2010.10.026

Wass CT, Lanier WL, Hofer RE, Scheithauer BW, Andrews AG (1995) Temperature changes of > or = 1 degree C alter functional neurologic outcome and histopathology in a canine model of complete cerebral ischemia. *Anesthesiology* 83(2): 325–335. doi: http://dx.doi.org/10.1097/00000542-199508000-00013

Whitelaw A, Thoresen M (2000) Antenatal steroids and the developing brain. *Arch Dis Child Fetal Neonatal Ed* 83(2): F154–F157. doi: http://dx.doi.org/10.1136/fn.83.2.f154

Wood C, Beard RW (1964) Temperature of the human foetus. *J Obstet Gynecol Br Commonw* 71: 768–769.

Wu YW, Escobar GJ, Grether JK, Croen LA, Greene JD, Newman TB (2003) Chorioamnionitis and cerebral palsy in term and near-term infants. *JAMA* 290(20): 2677–2684. doi: http://dx.doi.org/10.1001/jama.290.20.2677

Yoon BH, Jun JK, Romero R et al. (1997) Amniotic fluid inflammatory cytokines (interleukin-6, interleukin-1beta, and tumor necrosis factor-alpha), neonatal brain white matter lesions, and cerebral palsy. *Am J Obstet Gynecol* 177(1): 19–26. doi: http://dx.doi.org/10.1016/s0002-9378(97)70432-0

Yoon BH, Romero R, Park JS et al. (2000) Fetal exposure to an intra-amniotic inflammation and the development of cerebral palsy at the age of three years. *Am J Obstet Gynecol* 182(3): 675–681. doi: http://dx.doi.org/10.1067/mob.2000.104207

Yoon BH, Romero R, Yang SH et al. 1996. Interleukin-6 concentrations in umbilical cord plasma are elevated in neonates with white matter lesions associated with periventricular leukomalacia. *Am J Obstet Gynecol* 174(5): 1433–1440. doi: http://dx.doi.org/10.1016/s0002-9378(96)70585-9.

12
SUMMING-UP AND UNSOLVED PROBLEMS

Karin Nelson

The chapters in this book indicate that much is known about the role of the placenta, human or otherwise, in processes that are likely to be relevant to fetal brain development, but a great deal remains uncertain. As the next steps to increasing our understanding of the relationship of the placenta and congenital neurological disability become clearer, consideration of these main areas concludes this volume.

Development and function of the placenta

VASCULAR

The establishment of vascular connections between the fetus and mother via the placenta, arguably the most important feature of the human placenta, is described in Chapter 4. Information about this developing anatomy and factors that influence blood flow once the vasculature is established are critical for an understanding of much that follows, both in terms of placental and fetal outcomes.

A topic that is a dominant theme is the importance of fetal growth restriction (FGR) to neurological outcome. There exists a mechanism of FGR related to system A amino acid transporter activity, but pregnancy diseases are multifactorial and there are many potential causes of FGR: maternal, fetal and placental in origin.

ENDOCRINE

Although often described as providing a history or diary of pregnancy, the placenta is far more than a passive participant in the development of a new human being. (see Chapter 3). From the first days after fertilization the placenta produces humoral agents that (1) influence the uterus, (2) assume progesterone production from maternal corpus luteum and (3) influence the maternal hypothalamus. The placenta also liberates substances that impact on the fetal brain, producing serotonin for the forebrain before autonomous production in that locus (Bonnin and Levitt 2012), at a period when serotonin is a neurotrophic factor rather than a neurotransmitter.

Placental hormones influence a range of reproduction-relevant behaviors in the mother, including the familiar lassitude of early pregnancy. "Maternal feeding, maternal care, parturition, milk letdown and the suspension of fertility and sexual behaviour, are all determined by the maternal hypothalamus and have evolved to meet fetal needs under the influence of placental hormones" (Keverne 2012, p. 207). Maternal stress responses, in turn, alter brain development in the fetus via epigenetic mechanisms and DNA methylation (as specified in Chapter 10). These events are highly correlated between the placenta and fetal cortex (Jensen Pena et al. 2012).

Corticotrophins synthesized in the placenta are released in dramatically increasing amounts over the course of pregnancy and play a role in initiating labor and in modulating glucose transporter proteins in the placenta (Thomson 2013). Other examples of endocrine function of the placenta that relate to fetal brain development involve allopregnanalone and thyroid hormone (see Chapter 9).

As the work by Bonnin and Levitt (2012) on serotonin and the fetal forebrain makes clear, it is a task for the future to align the unfolding development of the brain to examine their interaction with processes in placental (patho) physiology. Although in this context, seemingly still early in the investigation of endocrine functions of the placenta, their role in fetal brain development promises to be an exciting topic for the future.

Pathogenic processes in the placenta which affect fetal brain

INFLAMMATION

Immunological function in pregnancy and its changes with gestational age, alongside outcomes in the child associated with intrauterine exposure to infection are discussed in relation to inflammation (see Chapters 5 and 6). It was reported in 1955 that maternal fever in labor is associated with heightened risk of cerebral palsy (CP) (Eastman and de Leon 1955) and since 1990 that a clinical diagnosis of chorioamnionitis, as well as maternal fever in labor, are risk factors for CP in infants of normal birthweight (Grether and Nelson 1997). Although these observations were described in total or in term and near-term infants, with 4.8% of CP patients associated with infant markers of inflammation (McIntyre et al. 2013), it is equally evident that the impact of intrauterine exposure to infection is marked in preterm infants, being a cause of both preterm birth and brain pathology in infants born too early.

INFECTION

Chorioamnionitis, of maternal involvement and funisitis, of fetal involvement, are infectious processes caused by specific micro-organisms differing in populations at different gestational ages. Viral infections in utero may also affect the fetus. Study has been chiefly in preterm neonates in which infection is a common cause of preterm birth. In these pregnancies, inflammatory placental lesions predominate, while, with increasing gestational age, vascular lesions become more prominent (Hecht et al. 2008). At the upper range of gestational ages, a population-based study of placental histology in stillbirths observed an increase in the frequency of chorioamnionitis and fetal response (Gordon et al. 2011), implying that developmental stage may strongly influence the impact of maternal inflammation upon the fetal brain (Carpentier et al. 2013).

Most observations concerning maternal infection and neurological outcome relate to infections identified during admission for delivery. However, maternal infection during pregnancy is also associated with a modest increase in the risk of CP (Miller et al. 2013).

Specific to the placenta, the multicentered Extremely Low Gestational Age Newborn (ELGAN) study (outlined in Chapter 6) has, for the first time, provided solid and welcome evidence that brain damage in extremely preterm infants is associated with microorganisms in the placenta parenchyma (O'Shea et al. 2009, Leviton 2010). In addition to defining a potential initiator of brain damage in these infants, the ongoing goal of this study is to better understand and thus clinically combat, the modulators, growth factors and other molecules that beget white matter damage in neonates. Within the ELGAN study, cytokine levels correlate with the nature of the condition leading to preterm birth (McElrath et al. 2011), supporting the concept that inflammation in very preterm infants is the result of antecedent conditions.

STERILE INFLAMMATION

Defined by areas of mononuclear cells in villous stroma, chronic villitis is fairly common in placentas at term. While noted in [T]oxoplasmosis, [O]ther Agents, [R]ubella, [C]ytomegalovirus and [H]erpes simplex; (TORCH infections (perinatal infections passed from mother to child), most villitis of unknown etiology (VUE) is thought to represent a breakdown of maternal tolerance of the feto-placental unit near term. VUE is associated with a number of risk factors for neonatal and hypoxic-ischemic encephalopathy (NE/HIE) and for CP, including prior pregnancy loss, FGR, abnormal fetal heart rate patterns, emergency surgical delivery and marked acidosis in the absence of sentinel events (McDonald et al. 2004, Redline 2007, Greer et al. 2012, Hayes et al. 2013). These features make it easy to confuse VUE with birth asphyxia and the distinction cannot be made without thorough placental examination. Indeed, neuroimaging evidence of lesions of basal ganglia and thalamus commonly attributed to birth asphyxia are also associated with VUE in NE/HIE patients (Hartemann et al. 2013).

So why is it important to recognize when neonatal neurological depression and acidosis occur in infants with placental VUE? First, there is no evidence that neonates whose neurological depression is related to VUE (or to infection) benefit from therapeutic hypothermia, a topic that calls for further investigation. Second, for those with VUE, benefit might be derived from therapies directed at the inflammatory process. Thus, placental examination to establish the presence of chorioamnionitis or funisitis or VUE may hold clinical importance for diagnosis and interpretation of trials of neonatal neuro-protective interventions.

HYPOXIA–ISCHEMIA

With modern obstetric care, hypoxia and ischemia probably play a less prominent role in the etiology of developmental disorders than in earlier times. In a population-based study, potential asphyxial birth events were associated with a doubling of risk for CP (OR 1.9) (CI 1.1–3.2) (McIntyre et al. 2013) alongside a higher risk of intrapartum stillbirth and neonatal hypoxic-ischemic encephalopathy. Thus, obstetric catastrophes remain important challenges for medical caregivers and the question is how to minimize their impact without compromising more mother–infant pairs that are benefitted.

Combined hypoxia–ischemia and inflammation increase the risk of perinatal brain injury. Fortunately, this combination is uncommon and accounts for less than 1% of all CP.

141

In comparison, the presence of both FGR and birth defects, recognized by early childhood, accounts for 8% of CP (McIntyre et al. 2013). Therefore, for prevention of congenital neurological disability, the focus of perinatal medicine should be broadened to include major contributors of risk other than hypoxia–ischemia. In this regard, evidence of vascular and inflammatory involvement, investigated through histologic and functional evaluations of the placenta and on brain and somatic maldevelopment, will eventually impact on clinical management and research.

FETAL GROWTH RESTRICTION

FGR is a risk factor for perinatal death and for a whole range of adverse neurological outcomes, neonatal and long-term (neonatal neurological depression, encephalopathy, perinatal stroke, CP, epilepsy, intellectual disability, autism and schizophrenia) and for other threats to health that may not be recognized until decades after birth (cardiovascular disease, diabetes, etc.). FGR is itself etiologically diverse, much of it having to do—as stressed in this volume—with factors that influence the production and transport of nutrients. Factors that coordinate nutrient supply in the placenta, matching demand to availability, such as mammalian target of rapamycin (mTOR), may play a role. In addition, mTOR is relevant to neurological development, at least in certain disorders, such as tuberous sclerosis and perhaps in seizure disorders more broadly.

Some conditions may lead to poor growth even when nutritional status is sufficient, such as TORCH and other infections. Still little explored is the association of low socio-economic status with risk of FGR (Ball et al. 2013) and of neonatal encephalopathy (Badawi et al. 1998, Blume et al. 2007). Whether recent discussions of the neurobiology underlying socio-economic differences in neurological outcome (Neville et al. 2013) are relevant here remains to be determined.

It is often assumed that the route from FGR to CP is via increased vulnerability of the growth-compromised fetus to the rigors of birth. However, large population-based studies have observed that asphyxial events at birth, leading to CP, are not more frequent in growth-restricted neonates than those of appropriate biometry (Blair et al. 2011, Stoknes et al. 2012). It therefore seems necessary in future studies of FGR outcome and intervention to consider subgroups of early and late-onset growth restriction with and without slow head growth, with and without congenital anomalies, as well as identifying specific syndromes of abnormal fetal growth in which their natural history antecedents clinical information (such as Doppler studies or magnetic resonance imaging) and placental findings are included. Defining etiological sub-syndromes of FGR will allow delineation of pathways related to fetal brain development, providing endophenotypes for genetic investigation and encourage further research in metabolic, toxic and other disorders that threaten neurological status, as well as a predisposition to disordered fetal growth.

ANIMAL MODELS OF FETAL GROWTH RESTRICTION

Although it is feasible to construct in utero animal models of FGR based upon specific etiologic factors, such as specific infections, nutritional deficits, toxic exposures, or perfusion insufficiencies, it is far more difficult to propose a convincing model that tests hypotheses of causation. Most observations of the human placenta in infants with encepha-lopathy reveal placental pathology, a fact requiring translation into animal simulations. However, placental types differ markedly (and perhaps relevantly) across species. The most common placental lesion in non-hypertensive FGR is chronic villitis (Pinar et al. 2011), which is chiefly an immunological lesion. It is not clear that a convincing animal model is yet available which reflects the complex disorders that afflict the majority of with encepha-lopathy human neonates and their placentas.

In a large population-based study, the majority of neonates with FGR who developed CP also had a birth defect recognized by early childhood (McIntyre et al. 2013). Thus, experimental models of exposures that can reproduce both restricted fetal growth and con-genital malformations are of special importance. It is likely that future experimental studies will address the impact of specific genomic abnormalities.

Cerebro-therapeutics
In considering the effects of perinatal interventions, (see Chapter 11) it may be desir-able to focus on the results of randomized-controlled clinical trials. One of the few perinatal interventions repeatedly demonstrated in well-conducted randomized trials to prevent CP and to qualify as primary prevention, is the antenatal administration of magnesium sulfate to women in very preterm labor (Gibbins et al. 2013). Although efficacy has been demonstrated with magnesium administration at later gestations, this has not been thoroughly tested (Nguyen et al. 2013). For secondary prevention in term and near-term infants, there is neonatal therapeutic hypothermia (Jacobs et al. 2013). This approach in neurologically depressed and acidotic term infants reduces the risk of CP, constituting secondary prevention, but it benefits only a minority of treated infants (Jacobs et al. 2013).

Antenatal corticosteroids improve survival and pulmonary function but are not shown to decrease neurological adversity, while postnatal dexamethasone threatens neurological integrity (Baud and Sola 2007).

In alternative approaches, administration of folate in pregnancy reduces the frequency of neural tube lesions, another success in primary prevention (Copp et al. 2013). Para-doxically, antibiotics in preterm deliveries may increase and not reduce vulnerability to CP (Kenyon et al. 2008). Identifying important risk factors for adverse neurological outcome does not necessarily guarantee that interventions directed at those factors will avert the unfortunate conclusion. As indicated in Chapter 5, while periodontal disease is associated with a heightened risk of preterm birth, its treatment fails to prevent it (or its adverse neurological consequences). In regard to preterm birth and placental abruptions, as these and presumably other overt complications are preceded by earlier in utero com-plications, which underscore the intertwined nature of aberrations in growth and neuro-logical development, the prevention of one antecedent may not offer the desired neuro-protective effects (Ananth and Wilcox 2001, Basso and Wilcox 2011), Some suc-cesses (as documented in Chapter 11) have been made, but clinical and research efforts must continue to seek strategies for prevention or amelioration of lifelong neurological disabilities of pre- and perinatal origin.

Placenta and neurological outcomes

Relating what is known of placental histopathology to clinical disorders producing developmental disabilities, is key in a volume on placental–clinical relationships (see Chapter 1). Redline ties together a variety of histologic lesions in the human placenta with birth outcome. In these endeavors, his own contribution has been enormous and he has been among the first investigators to quantify the specific features of placental histology—location, severity, chronicity—that influence the strength of association of specific histologic features and clinical consequences. In general, the neurological disorders in which placental abnormalities, macroscopic and/or histologic, have been reported are neonatal encephalopathy/HIE, neonatal seizures and CP. It is difficult to doubt the relevance of placental pathobiology to neurological outcome in antenatal and perinatal disorders and strong hypotheses have emerged. However, quantification and validation of these hypotheses are hampered by certain problems set before us.

Unsolved problems and what is needed

PROBLEMS IN CLINICAL-PATHOLOGICAL CORRELATIONS

The literature that seeks to connect placental features to clinical outcome in the child—even outcomes manifest in the newborn infant—is still sparse. As of this writing, for example, there are no controlled studies of placental pathology in perinatal stroke or in neonatal seizures and only a few in neonatal encephalopathy/HIE. Although different subtypes of CP can have different mechanisms, the only controlled and systematic investigation of placental findings in these is the ELGAN study, a single large multifaceted study of neonates of extremely low gestational age (O'Shea et al. 2009).

Aside from this study, the methodological quality in much of the literature is suboptimal. It is an important hurdle that most developmental disabilities cannot be diagnosed until months or years after birth, long after most placentas have been discarded. Studies are therefore difficult and seldom undertaken. Most available clinical-pathological studies to date are at the case series level, often uncontrolled or with participants who may not be typical of the general population.

Much of this volume on neurological outcome in association with placental findings examines relationships with CP. Why not a broader spectrum of outcomes, especially cognitive and psychiatric outcomes? The answer is that studies relating the placenta or birth events, or other biological risk factors, to intellectual or psychiatric outcomes require knowledge of the other major risk factors for these conditions. The strongest predictors of cognitive and psychiatric outcomes are socio-economic status and other characteristics of families that are seldom taken fully into account in perinatal studies. Without controls that consider these powerful determinants, studies of cognitive and psychiatric outcomes can be un-interpretable or misleading.

Existing studies relating placental histology to outcome have provided richly detailed descriptions of placental histologic findings, or provided well-characterized neurological outcomes; few studies provide expert classification of both placental features and neurological outcomes simultaneously. Although several systems for sampling, terminology and interpretation of placental histopathology have been proposed, none has achieved universal acceptance. Studies of inter-observer reliability suggest that specialized perinatal pathologists are in reasonable agreement with community pathologists in finding and describing chorioamnionitis, but confidence seems less justified about agreement in identifying other kinds of lesions (Grether et al. 1999, Simmonds et al. 2004, Redline et al. 2004). To assist, Pinar et al. (2011), in a large National Institute of Child Health and Human Development (NICHD)-supported study of stillborn infants and liveborn controls, have developed algorithms for describing placental lesions, rather than naming the lesions *per se*. This approach could eventually lead to computerized reading of placental histology, as currently performed for cervical (Pap) smears.

Interpretation of observations remains another source of potential uncertainty. When a specific placental lesion is observed in an individual with adverse outcome, or in a series of individuals, how sure is it that that lesion is causal or contributory to the unsatisfactory outcome? A number of questions arise, including the lesions' location, number, severity, duration and whether other potentially relevant kinds of lesions are also present. Whether and when a placental histologic condition can be considered causal or contributory can only be answered by a series of large controlled studies in representative populations, in which the magnitude of outcome risk is identified in combination with the presence of the specific lesion. Such studies have yet to be performed.

With regard to follow-up studies, no contemporary longitudinal investigations connect maternal and family history, pregnancy and delivery history, placental findings (histologic and functional), nursery course (neonatal intensive care, etc.) and long-term outcome in term and late preterm infants. Consequently, the natural history of placental disease remains very incomplete and potential opportunities for clinical intervention remain unidentified. Incorporation of imaging of placenta and of fetal or neonatal brain, biomarkers including those examined by multiplex platforms of neonatal/maternal samples and contemporaneous genetic/genomic technologies will undoubtedly have future roles in addressing these shortfalls.

What is needed?

Examples of approaches that may be feasible in some settings are routine placental examination performed by standardized study design in specific high-risk situations—all placentas of term infants requiring respiratory support at 10 minutes of life, for example, or all those who are found to be markedly growth restricted on delivery, with specified collection of control placentas of neonates of similar sex and gestational age. Performance of such studies in regions that have CP and birth defects registries would maximize information and minimize cost. Inclusion of placental examination in randomized trials of perinatal neuroprotection, with secondary analysis stratified on placental findings and other clinical data collected after randomization, would permit an expanded understanding of the situations in which therapeutic hypothermia, for example, is most helpful and perhaps identify etiological subgroups in which cooling fails to benefit neonates.

Conclusion

As exemplified in this book, much is now known relating the placenta to fetal brain development, be it normal or abnormal, but much remains undescribed. Where obstetric care is good, hypoxia–ischemia is no longer a dominant cause of neurodisability, but the roles of other causal factors remain under-explored. Much is yet to be learned about inflammation (infectious and immunologic), aberrations of fetal growth and of birth defects and the role of genetic and environmental factors in neurodisability. Longitudinal studies in humans are needed that allow delineation of disorders with FGR as a prominent feature and of placental inflammation, relating developmental disabilities and placental and other information to that natural history.

Two conditions of high risk for neurodisability are recognizable in the delivery room, before placentas have been discarded: neonatal encephalopathy/HIE and FGR. A focus on collecting placentas of such infants and conducting follow-up studies of these and control children will be important steps in understanding the relationship of the human placenta and fetal brain development and its aberrations. Furthermore, placental–clinical correlative studies will be important in the future of fetal and perinatal medicine and in the understanding of the biological foundation of many forms of congenital neurological disability.

As stated by Zeltser and Leibel (2011), "together [current] studies suggest that the traditional view of the placenta as a passive site of transport of maternal nutrients, growth factors and hormones needs to be expanded to include a role in supporting CNS development through adaptive responses to the maternal environment" (p. 15667).

REFERENCES

Ananth CV, Wilcox AJ (2001) Placental abruption and perinatal mortality in the United States. *Am J Epidemiol* 153(4): 332–337. doi: http://dx.doi.org/10.1093/aje/153.4.332.

Badawi N, Kurinczuk JJ, Keogh JM et al. (1998) Antepartum risk factors for newborn encephalopathy: The Western Australian case-control study. *BMJ* 317(7172): 1549–1553. doi: http://dx.doi.org/10.1136/bmj.317.7172.1549.

Ball SJ, Jacoby P, Zubrik SR (2013) Socioeconomic status accounts for rapidly increasing geographic variation in the incidence of poor fetal growth. *Int J Environ Res Public Health* 10(7): 2606–2620. doi: http://dx.doi.org/10.3390/ijerph10072606.

Basso O, Wilcox AJ (2011) Might rare factors account for most of the mortality of preterm babies? *Epidemiology* 22(3): 320–327. doi: http://dx.doi.org/10.1097/EDE.0b013e31821266c5.

Baud O, Sola A (2007) Corticosteroids in perinatal medicine: How to improve outcomes without affecting the developing brain? *Semin Fetal Neonatal Med* 12(4): 273–279. doi: http://dx.doi.org/10.1016/j.siny.2007.01.025.

Blair E, de Groot J, Nelson KB (2011) Placental infarction identified by macroscopic examination and risk of cerebral palsy in infants at 35 weeks of gestational age and over. *Am J Obstet Gynecol* 205: 124.e1–124.e7. doi: http://dx.doi.org/10.1016/j.ajog.2011.05.022.

Blume HK, Loch CM, Li CI (2007) Neonatal encephalopathy and socioeconomic status: Population-based casecontrol study. *Arch Pediatr Adolesc Med* 161(7): 663–668. doi: http://dx.doi.org/10.1001/archpedi.161.7.663.

Bonnin A, Levitt P (2012) Placental source for 5-HT that tunes fetal brain development. *Neuropsychopharmacology* 37(1): 299–300. doi: http://dx.doi.org/10.1038/npp.2011.194.

Carpentier PA, Haditsch U, Braun AE et al. (2013) Stereotypical alterations in cortical patterning are associated with maternal illness-induced placental dysfunction. *J Neurosci* 33(43): 16874–1688. doi: http://dx.doi.org/10.1523/JNEUROSCI.4654-12.2013.

Copp AJ, Stanier P, Greene ND (2013) Neural tube defects: Recent advances, unsolved questions, and controversies. *Lancet Neurol* 12(8): 799–810. doi: http://dx.doi.org/10.1016/s1474-4422(13)70110-8.

Eastman NJ, DeLeon M (1955) The etiology of cerebral palsy. *Am J Obstet Gynecol* 69(5): 950–961.

Gibbins KJ, Browning KR, Lopes VV, Anderson BL, Rouse DJ (2013) Evaluation of the clinical use of magnesium sulfate for cerebral palsy prevention. *Obstet Gynecol* 121(2 Pt 1): 235–240.

Gordon A, Lahra M, Raynes-Greenow C, Jeffery H (2011) Histological chorioamnionitis is increased at extremes of gestation in stillbirth: A population-based study. *Infect Dis Obstet Gynecol* 2011: 1–7. doi: http://dx.doi.org/10.1155/2011/456728.

Greer LG, Ziadie MS, Casey BM, Rogers BB, McIntire DD, Leveno KJ (2012) An immunologic basis for placental insufficiency in fetal growth restriction. *Am J Perinatol* 29(7): 533–538. doi: http://dx.doi.org/10.1055/s-0032-1310525.

Grether JK, Eaton A, Redline R, Bendon R, Benirschke K, Nelson K (1999) Reliability of placental histology using archived specimens. *Paediatr Perinat Epidemiol* 13(4): 489–495. doi: http://dx.doi.org/10.1046/j.1365-3016.1999.00214.x.

Grether JK, Nelson KB (1997) Maternal infection and cerebral palsy in infants of normal birth weight. *JAMA* 278(3): 207–211. Erratum in: (1998) *JAMA* 279(2): 118. doi: http://dx.doi.org/10.1001/jama.1997.03550030047032.

Hartemann JC, Nikkels PG, Benders MJ, Kwee A, Groenendaal F, de Vries LS (2013) Placental pathology in fullterm infants with hypoxic-ischemic neonatal encephalopathy and association with magnetic resonance imaging pattern of brain injury. *J Pediatr* 163(4): 968–975.e2. doi: http://dx.doi.org/10.1016/j.jpeds.2013.06.010.

Hayes BC, Cooley S, Donnelly E et al. (2013) The placenta in infants >=36 weeks gestation with neonatal encephalopathy: A case control study. *Arch Dis Child Fetal Neonatal Ed* 98(3): F233–F239. doi: http://dx.doi.org/10.1136/archdischild-2012-301992.

Hecht JL, Allred EN, Kliman HJ et al. (2008) Histological characteristics of singleton placentas delivered before the 28th week of gestation. *Pathology* 40(4): 372–376. doi: http://dx.doi.org/10.1080/00313020802035865. PMID: 18446627.

Jacobs SE, Berg M, Hunt R, Tarnow-Mordi WO, Inder TE, Davi PG (2013) Cooling for newborns with hypoxic ischaemic encephalopathy. *Cochrane Database Syst Rev* 1: CD003311. doi: http://dx.doi.org/10.1002/14651858.CD003311.pub3.

Jensen Pena C, Monk C, Champagne FA (2012) Epigenetic effects of prenatal stress on 11 -hydroxysteroid dehydrogenase-2 in the placenta and fetal brain. *PLoS ONE* 7(6): e39791. doi: http://dx.doi.org/10.1371/journal.pone.0039791.

Kenyon S, Brocklehurst P, Jones D, Marlow N, Salt A, Taylor D (2008) MRC ORACLE Children Study. Long term outcomes following prescription of antibiotics to pregnant women with either spontaneous preterm labour or preterm rupture of the membranes. *BMC Pregnancy Childbirth* 8: 14. doi: http://dx.doi.org/10.1186/1471-2393-8-14.

Keverne EB (2012) Significance of epigenetics for understanding brain development, brain evolution and behaviour. *Neuroscience*. doi:pii: S0306-4522(12)01141-4. doi: http://dx.doi.org/10.1016/j.neuroscience.2012.11.030.

Leviton A, Allred EH, Kuban KC et al. (2010) Microbiologic and histologic characteristics of the extremely preterm infant's placenta predict white matter damage and later cerebral palsy: The ELGAN study. *Pediatr Res* 67(1): 95–101. doi: http://dx.doi.org/10.1203/pdr.0b013e3181bf5fab.

Loke YW (2013) *Life's vital link: The astonishing role of the placenta.* Oxford, UK Oxford University Press.

McDonald DG, Kelehan P, McMenamin JB (2004) Placental fetal thrombotic vasculopathy is associated with neonatal encephalopathy. *Hum Pathol* 35(7): 875–880. doi: http://dx.doi.org/10.1016/j.humpath.2004.02.014.

McElrath TF, Fichorova RN, Allred EN et al; ELGAN Study Investigators (2011) Blood protein profiles of infants born before 28 weeks differ by pregnancy complication. *Am J Obstet Gynecol* 204(5): 418.e1–418.e12. doi: http://dx.doi.org/10.1016/j.ajog.2010.12.010.

McIntyre S, Taitz D, Keogh J, Goldsmith S, Badawi N, Blair E (2013) A systematic review of risk factors for cerebral palsy in children born at term in developed countries. *Dev Med Child Neurol* 55(6): 499–508. doi: http://dx.doi.org/10.1111/dmcn.12017. Epub 2012 Nov 26.

Miller JE, Pedersen LH, Streja E et al. (2013) Maternal infections during pregnancy and cerebral palsy: A population-based cohort study. *Paediatr Perinat Epidemiol* 27(6): 542–552. doi: http://dx.doi.org/10.1111/ppe.12082.

Neville H, Stevens C, Pakulak E, Bell TA (2013) Commentary: Neurocognitive consequences of socioeconomic disparities. *Dev Sci* 16(5): 708–712. doi: http://dx.doi.org/10.1111/desc.12081.

Nguyen TM, Crowther CA, Wilkinson D, Bain E (2013) Magnesium sulphate for women at term for neuroprotection of the fetus. *Cochrane Database Syst Rev* 2: CD009395. doi: 10.1002/14651858.CD009395.pub2.

O'Shea TM, Allred EN, Dammann O et al; ELGAN study Investigators (2009) The ELGAN study of the brain and related disorders in extremely low gestational age newborns. *Early Hum Dev* 85(11): 719–725. doi: http://dx.doi.org/10.1016/j.earlhumdev.2009.08.060. Epub 2009 Sep 17.

Pinar H, Koch MA, Hawkins H et al. (2011) The Stillbirth Collaborative Research Network (SCRN) placental and umbilical cord examination protocol. *Am J Perinatol* 28(10): 781–792. doi: http://dx.doi.org/10.1055/s-0031-1281509.

Redline RW, Boyd T, Campbell V et al. (2004) Maternal vascular underperfusion: Nosology and reproducibility of placental reaction patterns. *Pediatr Dev Pathol* 7(3): 237–249. doi: http://dx.doi.org/10.1007/s10024-003-8083-2.

Redline RW (2007) Villitis of unknown etiology: Noninfectious chronic villitis in the placenta. *Hum Pathol* 38(10): 1439–1446. doi: http://dx.doi.org/10.1016/j.humpath.2007.05.025.

Simmonds M, Jeffery H, Watson G, Russell P (2004) Intraobserver and interobserver reliability for the histologic diagnosis of chorioamnionitis. *Am J Obstet Ggyn* 190(1): 152–155. doi: http://dx.doi.org/10.1016/s0002-9378(03)00870-6.

Stoknes M, Andersen GL, Dahlseng MO et al. (2012) Cerebral palsy and neonatal death in term singletons born small for gestational age. *Pediatrics* 130: e1629. doi: http://dx.doi.org/10.1542/peds.2012-0152.

Thomson M (2013) The physiological roles of placental corticotropin releasing hormone in pregnancy and childbirth. *J Physiol Biochem* 69(3): 559–573. doi: http://dx.doi.org/10.1007/s13105-012-0227-2.

Zeltser LM, Leibel RL (2011) Roles of the placenta in fetal brain development. *Proc Natl Acad Sci* 108(38): 15667–15668. Doi: http://dx.doi.org/10.1073/pnas.1112239108.

INDEX

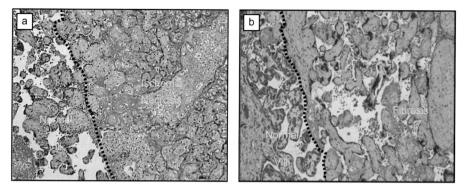

Fig. 1.2. (p 5) Placental vascular lesions with high prevalence in neonatal brain injury. (a) Maternal villous infarct: A portion of the distal villous tree shows ischemic necrosis of villous trophoblast and obliteration of the intervillous space, secondary to obstruction of a maternal spiral artery. Villous stromal and vascular architecture is preserved. Normal villi are seen on the left (H&E stain, 10x magnification). (b) Fetal thrombotic vasculopathy: A portion of the distal villous tree shows loss of fetal vessels and stromal fibrosis secondary to obstruction of a large fetal placental vessel. Villous trophoblast and intervillous space are preserved. Normal villi seen on the left side (H&E stain, 10x magnification).

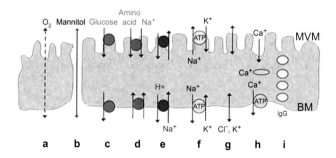

Fig. 2.2. (p 12) Schematic diagram of the major mechanisms of transfer across the placental microvillous membrane (MVM) and basal membrane (BPM) of the syncytiotrophoblast: (a) simple diffusion of relatively lipophilic substances; (b) paracellular route for hydrophilic substances: (c–h) transporter-mediated transport: (c) facilitated diffusion; (d) co-transport; (e) exchange; and (f,h) active transport. ATP; adenosine triphosphate. Ion channels (g,h) are present in the MVM and BPM and there is evidence for endocytosis–exocytosis (i). Examples of solutes transported by each mechanism are included. Reproduced from *Int J Dev Biol* (2010) 54: 377–390 with permission from University of the Basque Country Press.

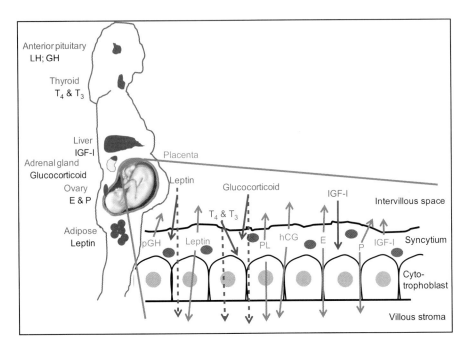

Fig. 3.1. (p 23) Maternal and placental production of hormones regulating placental and fetal growth. Maternal hormones and their sites of production are shown in red. Solid red arrows indicate action in placenta, whereas dotted red arrows denote hormones that are transferred across the placenta into the fetal circulation. Hormones produced by the placenta are shown in blue; all have functions within the placenta and their secretion into the maternal and fetal circulations is depicted by blue arrows.

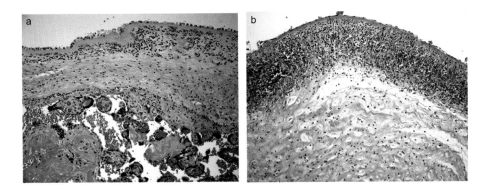

Fig. 6.1. (p 62) Histological sections of fetal membranes showing inflammatory infiltrate (blue polymorphonuclear leukocytes) characteristic of severe chorioamnionitis. (a) Neutrophils migrating toward the amniotic cavity. (b) Necrotizing chorioamnionitis characterized by severe acute inflammation and focal necrosis. Reproduced from *Surg Pathol Clin: Placental Pathol* 6 (1): 33–60, with permission from WB Saunders.

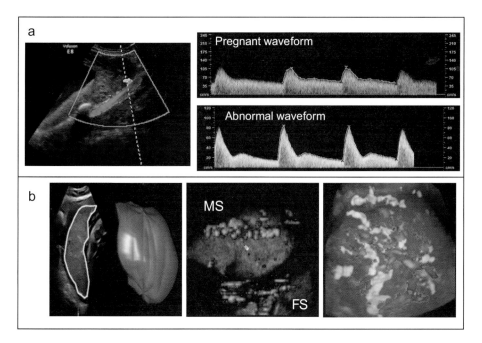

Fig. 8.1. (p 85) Ultrasound investigations of the utero-placenta. (a) Identification and Doppler waveform of the uterine artery. Abnormal placentation characterised by elevated resistance and retained early diastolic notch. (b) 3D ultrasound showing volume determination of the placenta and power Doppler rendering of placental blood flow on the placental chorionic (fetal side FS) and basal plate (maternal side MS).

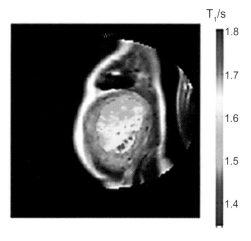

Fig. 8.3. (p 89) Placental MRI map showing sensitivity to oxygen saturation (PO_2). T1-weight image obtained in an in-plane view superimposed on a T2-weighted structural image.

155

Recent titles from Mac Keith Press www.mackeith.co.uk

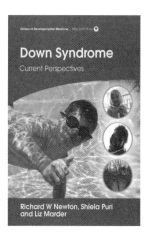

Down Syndrome: Current Perspectives
Richard W Newton, Shiela Puri and Liz Marder (Editors)

Clinics in Developmental Medicine
2015 ▪ 320pp ▪ hardback ▪ 978-1-909962-47-7
£95.00 / €118.00 / $150.00

Down syndrome remains the most common recognisable form of intellectual disability. The challenge for doctors today is how to capture the rapidly expanding body of scientific knowledge and devise models of care to meet the needs of individuals and their families. *Down Syndrome: Current Perspectives* provides doctors and other health professionals with the information they need to address the challenges that can present in the management of syndrome.

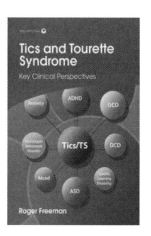

Tics and Tourette Syndrome: Key Clinical Perspectives
Roger Freeman

2015▪ 304pp ▪ softback ▪ 978-1-909962-41-5
£55.95/ €72.95 / $90.00

Written by a world-renowned expert in developmental neurology, this book will be of practical use to clinicians who may encounter tic disorders and Tourette syndrome that complicate the management of their patients. It contains wide-ranging discussion of tics that occur alone or in other conditions such as ADHD, DCD, and ASD. It includes extensive information on stereotypic movement disorder and other repetitive movements which are often confused with tics.

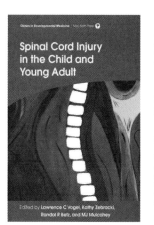

Spinal Cord Injury in the Child and Young Adult
Lawrence C Vogel, Kathy Zebracki, Randall R Betz and MJ Mulcahey (Editors)

Clinics in Developmental Medicine
2014 ▪ 460pp ▪ hardback ▪ 978-1-909962-34-7
£125.00 / €155.10 / $206.50

Compared to adult-onset spinal cord injury (SCI), individuals with childhood-onset SCI are unique in several ways. As a result of their younger age at injury and longer lifespan, individuals with paediatric-onset SCI are particularly susceptible to long-term complications related to a sedentary lifestyle. This book is intended for clinicians of all disciplines who may only occasionally care for young people with SCI to those who specialize in SCI as well as clinical and basic researchers in the SCI field.

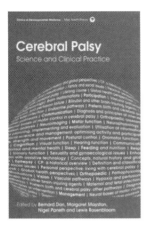

Cerebral Palsy: Science and Clinical Practice
Bernard Dan, Margaret Mayston, Nigel Paneth
and Lewis Rosenbloom (Editors)

Clinics in Developmental Medicine
2014 ▪ 712pp ▪ hardback ▪ 978-1-909962-38-5
£190.00 / €235.80 / $299.95

The only complete, scientifically rigorous, fully integrated reference giving a wide-ranging and in-depth perspective on cerebral palsy and related neurodevelopment disabilities. It considers all aspects of cerebral palsy from the causes to clinical problems and their implications for individuals. Leading scientists present the evidence on the role of preterm birth, inflammation, hypoxia, endocrinological and other pathways. They explore opportunities for neuroprotection leading to clinical applications.

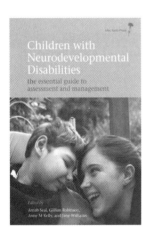

Children with Neurodevelopmental Disabilities: the essential guide to assessment and management
Arnab Seal, Gillian Robinson, Anne M. Kelly
and Jane Williams (Editors)

2013 ▪ 744pp ▪ softback ▪ 978-1-908316-62-2
£65.00 / €78.00 / $99.95

A comprehensive textbook on the practice of paediatric neurodisability, written by practitioners and experts in the field. Using a problem-oriented approach, the authors give best-practice guidance, and centre on the needs of the child and family, working in partnership with multi-disciplinary, multi-agency teams. It provides a ready reference for managing problems encountered in the paediatric clinic.

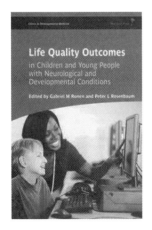

Life Quality Outcomes in Children and Young People with Neurological and Developmental Conditions
Gabriel M. Ronen and Peter L. Rosenbaum (Editors)

Clinics in Developmental Medicine
2013 ▪ 394pp ▪ hardback ▪ 978-1-908316-58-5
£95.00 / €120.70 / $149.95

Healthcare professionals need to understand their patients' views of their condition and its effects on their health and well-being. This book builds on the World Health Organization's concepts of 'health', 'functioning' and 'quality of life' for young people with neuro-disabilities; it emphasises the importance of engaging with patients in the identification of both treatment goals and their evaluation. Uniquely, it enables healthcare professionals to find critically reviewed outcomes-related information.

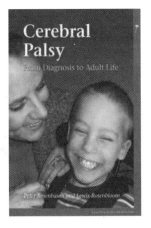

Cerebral Palsy: From Diagnosis to Adult Life
Peter L. Rosenbaum and Lewis Rosenbloom

A practical guide from Mac Keith Press
2012 ▪ 224pp ▪ softback ▪ 978-1-908316-50-9
£29.95 / €36.00 / $50.00

This book has been designed to provide readers with an understanding of cerebral palsy as a developmental as well as a neurological condition. It details the nature of cerebral palsy, its causes and its clinical manifestations. Using clear, accessible language (supported by an extensive glossary) the authors have blended current science with metaphor to explain the biomedical underpinnings of the disorder.

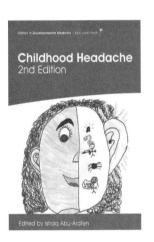

Childhood Headache, 2nd Edition
Ishaq Abu-Arafeh (Editor)

Clinics in Developmental Medicine
2013 ▪ 352pp ▪ hardback ▪ 978-1-908316-75-2
£95.00 / €115.20 / $154.95

Headache is a common problem which has a significant impact on children's quality of life. *Childhood Headache* is a comprehensive source of knowledge and guidance to practising clinicians looking after children with headache that includes many clinical examples to illustrate the difficulties in diagnosis or options for treatment. It is also a resource for researchers who are looking for a full analysis of the published studies.

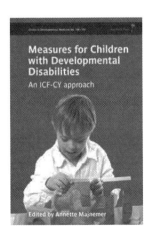

Measures for Children with Developmental Disabilities
An ICF-CY approach
Annette Majnemer (Editor)

linics in Developmental Medicine No 194-195
2012 ▪ 552pp ▪ hardback ▪ 978-1-908316-45-5
£154.00 / €184.80 / $235.00

This title presents and reviews outcome measures across a wide range of attributes that are applicable to children and adolescents with developmental disabilities. It uses the children and youth version of the International Classification of Functioning, Disability and Health (ICF-CY) as a framework for organizing the various measures into sections and chapters. Each chapter coincides with domains within the WHO framework of Body Functions, Activities and Participation, and Personal and Environmental Factors.

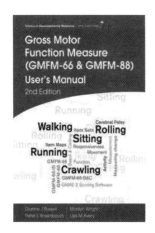

Gross Motor Function Measure (GMFM-66 and GMFM-88) User's Manual, 2nd Edition
Dianne J. Russell, Peter L. Rosenbaum, Marilyn Wright, Lisa M. Avery

Clinics in Developmental Medicine
2013 ▪ 304pp ▪ spiral-bound softback ▪ 978-1-908316-88-2
£70.00 / €84.00 / $115.00

The Gross Motor Function Measure (GMFM) has become the best evaluative measure of motor function designed for quantifying change in the gross motor abilities of children with cerebral palsy. The new version of the scoring programme has now been released, and includes two abbreviated methods of estimating GMFM-66 scores using the GMFM-66-Item sets and the GMFM-66-Basal & Ceiling. This new edition builds on the wide success of the first edition.

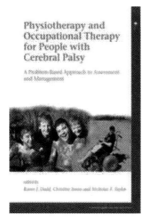

Physiotherapy and Occupational Therapy for People with Cerebral Palsy
Karen J. Dodd, Christine Imms, Nicholas F. Taylor (Editors)

A practical guide from Mac Keith Press
2010 ▪ 320pp ▪ softback ▪ 978-1-898683-68-1
£29.95/ €36.00 / $41.99
This book is a practical resource for physiotherapists and occupational therapists who support people with cerebral palsy, helping them to solve the problems with movement and other impairments that so often accompany cerebral palsy, so that they can be more active and better able to participate in roles such as study, work, recreation and relationships

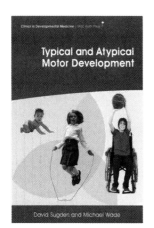

Typical and Atypical Motor Development
David Sugden and Michael Wade

Clinics in Developmental Medicine
2013 ▪ 400pp ▪ hardback ▪ 978-1-908316-55-4
£145.00 / €180.00 / $234.95

Sugden and Wade, leading authors in this area, comprehensively cover motor development and motor impairment, drawing on sources in medicine and health-related studies, motor learning and developmental psychology. A theme that runs through the book is that movement outcomes are a complex transaction of child resources, the context in which movement takes place, and the manner in which tasks are presented.